# THE GOOD LFE COOKBOOK

*low fermentation eating for SIBO, gut health, and microbiome balance*

*by Krystyna Houser & Robin Berlin, RDN*

## GOODL/FE
low fermentation eating

Good LFE is a multifaceted product and lifestyle brand focusing on microbiome health and wellness for those struggling with SIBO, IBS, and other gastrointestinal issues.

Founded by Dr. Mark Pimentel, Dr. Ali Rezaie, Robin Berlin RDN, and Krystyna Houser, all leading experts and voices in their fields.

Good LFE is the result of their desire to bring motivation and inspiration to the IBS, SIBO, and microbiome-conscious community.

Join us. Learn more at www.thegoodlfe.com and gain access to articles, videos, recipes, and more.

## AGATE

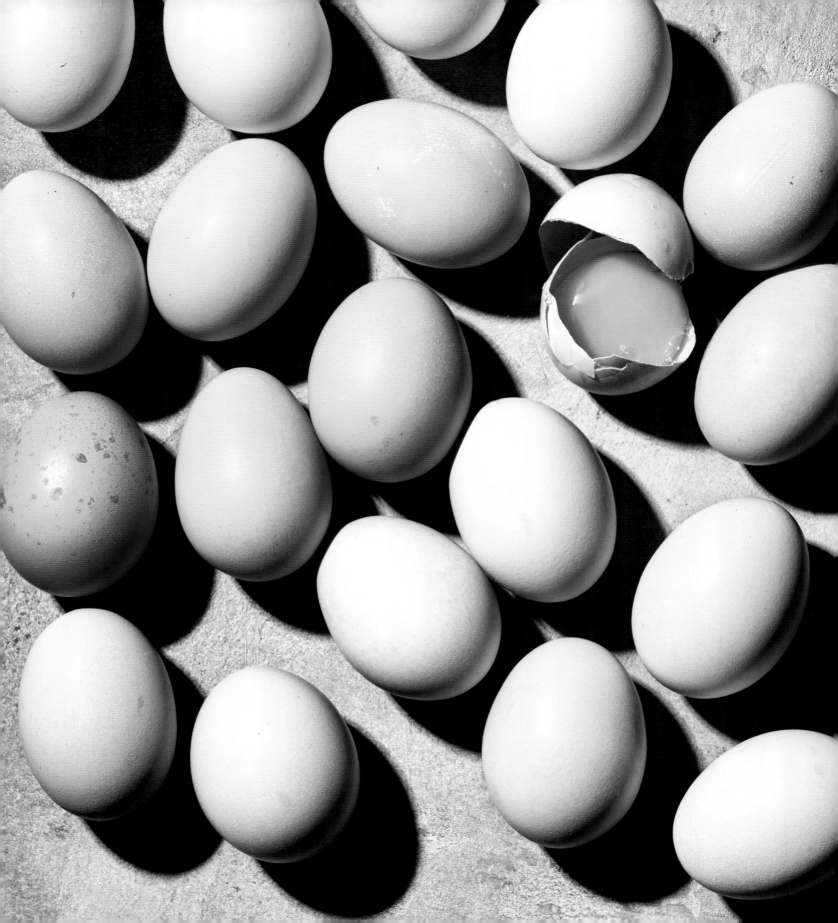

# CONTENTS

**LF | V | GF**
*Lactose-free, Vegan, Gluten-free*

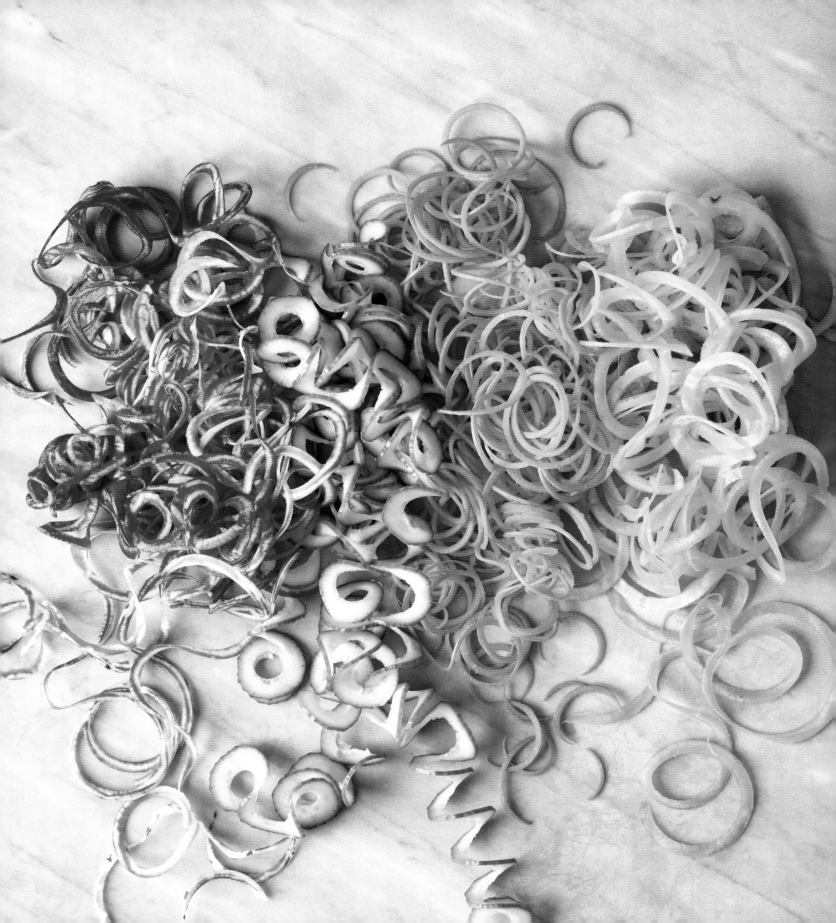

# FOREWORD / SIBO & MICROBIOME BALANCE BY DR. MARK PIMENTEL & DR. ALI REZAIE

We have spent decades researching and treating gastrointestinal issues, with a significant focus and expertise on the treatment of Small Intestinal Bacterial Overgrowth (SIBO) and microbiome health. Over time, we have demonstrated that the best way to restore microbiome balance and gut health is in fact through diet. As a result, we developed the Low Fermentation Eating (LFE) plan, upon which the Good LFE Cookbook is based.

Recent science suggests that humans are not *entirely* "human." Your gut is home to a cast of trillions of bacteria, viruses, and fungi. In fact, the number of bacterial cells in the human body exceeds the number of human cells in the body. These microbes can be beneficial, opportunistic, and at times, disease-causing. So every time you eat, you are sharing your meal with the vast array of microbes in the gut. For many people, food is simply absorbed in the small intestine and they go about their day. For those with SIBO, an excessive amount of bacteria have taken up residence in the small intestine where it can live off of fresh food, hence the name SIBO, Small Intestinal Bacterial Overgrowth.

While the complexity of this diagnosis is beyond this foreword, a hallmark of this disease is that people with SIBO have uncomfortable bloating after eating and in the more extreme cases stomach pain. Having SIBO creates a conundrum. You need a balanced diet to be healthy, but how do you do that when the bacteria of SIBO are there to ferment food and cause symptoms? Historically, extreme diets have been proposed but now we know these are too restrictive and unhealthy for you in the long run. Life cannot be about a daily struggle for diet. Eating is complex, and while there is no one perfect diet, years of scientific investigation and experience have taught us that experiencing SIBO or bloating involves two factors. First is how you eat—allow time between eating for the gut to clean itself in preparation for the next meal. And secondly, to eat in a way that is healthy with balanced nutrients, yet not too restrictive (so you can find food on a restaurant menu and enjoy life.)

Often, eating to restore microbiome balance can be restrictive, difficult, and bland, adding to the woes of a SIBO sufferer. This cookbook solves for this with flavorful, accessible meals that can bring the joy of eating back to those with gastrointestinal issues. And there is a secret here: these recipes taste good for everyone.

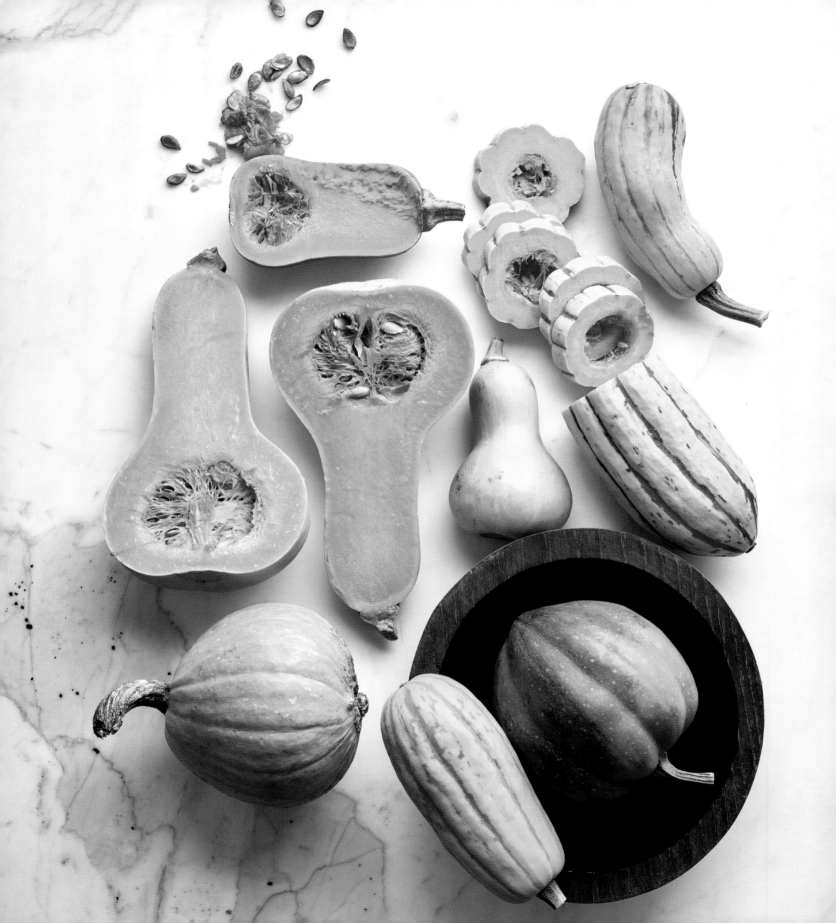

# HOW WE MADE IT HAPPEN

Creating this cookbook was a labor of love for us. We have both spent years trying to find microbiome balance, and this book represents a final step on that journey—sharing all that we have learned so that others can benefit from our experiences.

Getting this far has not always been easy. SIBO and other microbiome issues are usually poorly diagnosed or misdiagnosed several times, while symptoms, including the horrible cocktail of bloating and brain fog, get worse and worse. Certainly, that was true for both of us. As so many others experience, we were told for years that it was "all in our heads." It's not all in your head, it's all in your gut. And while the brain-gut connection isn't fully understood yet, it is well documented and very real. We understand because we have lived it.

It takes a little effort and organization to integrate eating for SIBO and microbiome balance into a life full of family, friends, work, and everything else, but the results have been spectacular—we have got our lives back. Despite the challenges of living with SIBO, we are grateful that this diagnosis brought us together and led to this cookbook. This is our first compilation about how to tweak foods we love to ensure they not only bring pleasure but also keep our microbiome in balance. It has taken a lot of fun experimentation, and more than one upturned nose as we first offered our families "new" versions of their favorites, and in the end we are incredibly proud of the results. Living with SIBO changed the rules for foods and ingredients but we were determined to find a way to love food again. The hard work paid off and now we can live each day feeling satisfied, not deprived, and SIBO-free. We remain optimistic that the right diet can radically improve anyone's microbiome, and believe in the connection that happens when we come together to share a meal.

## KRYSTYNA & ROBIN

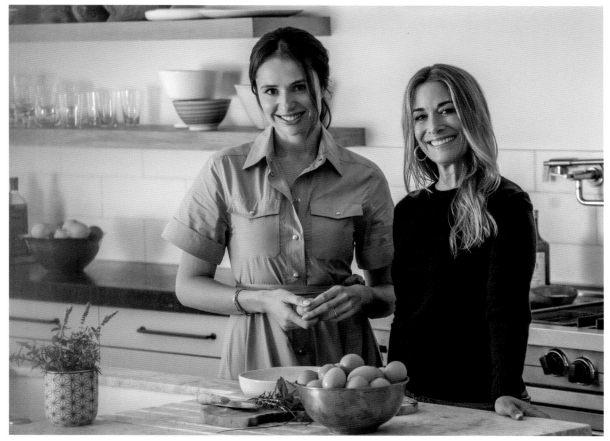

Photograph: Alex Freund

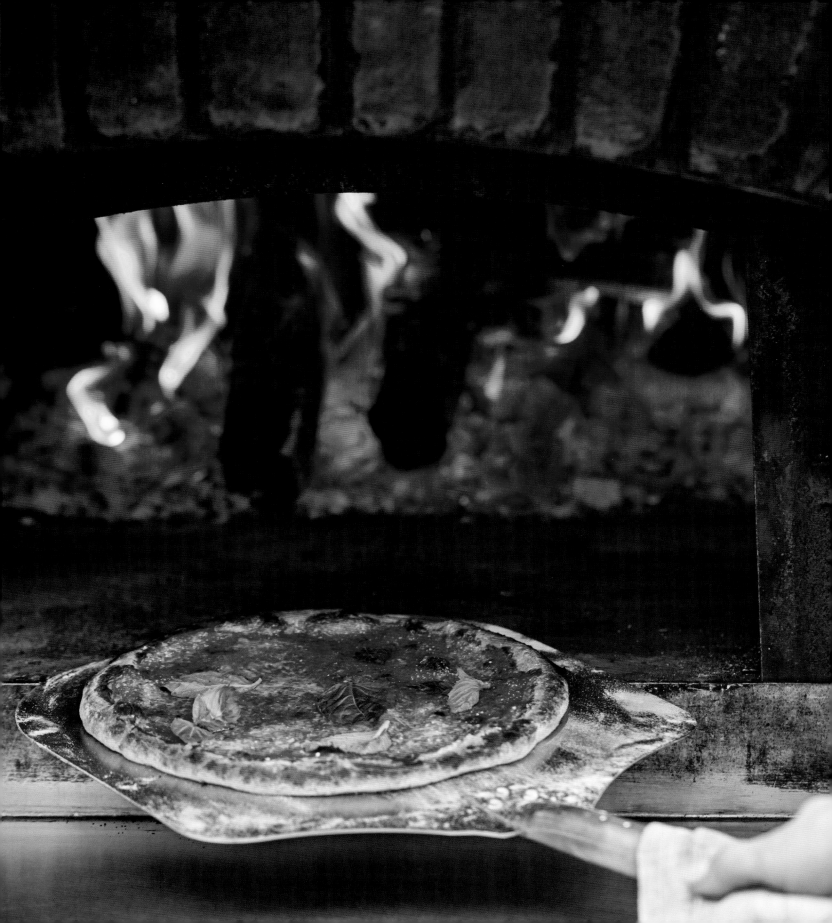

# INTRODUCTION

This book is a celebration of food and the joys of eating. Using fresh, seasonal ingredients, we show you how to simply cook delicious, flavorful meals to keep your microbiome healthy and balanced. Tapping into decades of gastrointestinal research, our recipes are based upon Low Fermentation Eating (LFE), and are designed to support a healthy gut environment. Building on family favorites, some handed down for generations, these recipes have been adjusted to make them SIBO-friendly, yet without sacrificing the flavors and textures that have put them on our tables day-after-day and season-after-season.

You will find a wide selection of recipes from satisfying weeknight meals to show-stopping dinners for celebrations. All the recipes, from the familiar spaghetti Bolognese to the more adventurous paella, were designed for the everyday cook. There are no complicated techniques to master—if you can chop a carrot, you can cook these meals. Every recipe in this book is SIBO-friendly and designed to help keep your microbiome in balance. (Of course, we recognize that every microbiome is different and have called out omissions or swaps around items that may trigger some people's systems but not others.)

This book is organized by seasons to maximize nutrition and simplify your life. When possible, we cook with seasonal vegetables and fruits so that we can enjoy them at their optimal levels of flavor and nutrition. Additionally, being able to use ingredients that are readily at hand also adds a level of convenience and simplicity. Every season includes recipes that will get you from breakfast to dinner, including drinks to help you unwind at the end of the day. We have organized them by meal—breakfast, lunch, dinner, etc.—but of course these are not hard and fast rules. We say listen to your body and if you are craving breakfast for dinner, enjoy. The only rules we believe in following are eating what makes both you, and your microbiome, happy. The recipes within each seasonal section also include solutions that meet the needs of that season—great brunch recipes for spring celebrations, lighter options for summer when mealtimes often push later and crowd-pleasing appetizers and mains for the hectic, entertaining holiday season.

We have worked to create a cookbook that opens up a world of flavorful eating for those with a SIBO diagnosis or other microbiome issues yet is also a great resource for anyone looking for delicious, healthy meals. We are overjoyed to be sharing the results with you and wish you well on your journey to microbiome health.

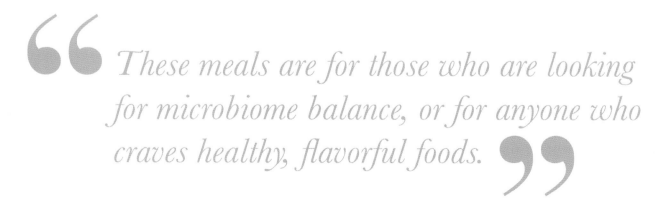

*These meals are for those who are looking for microbiome balance, or for anyone who craves healthy, flavorful foods.*

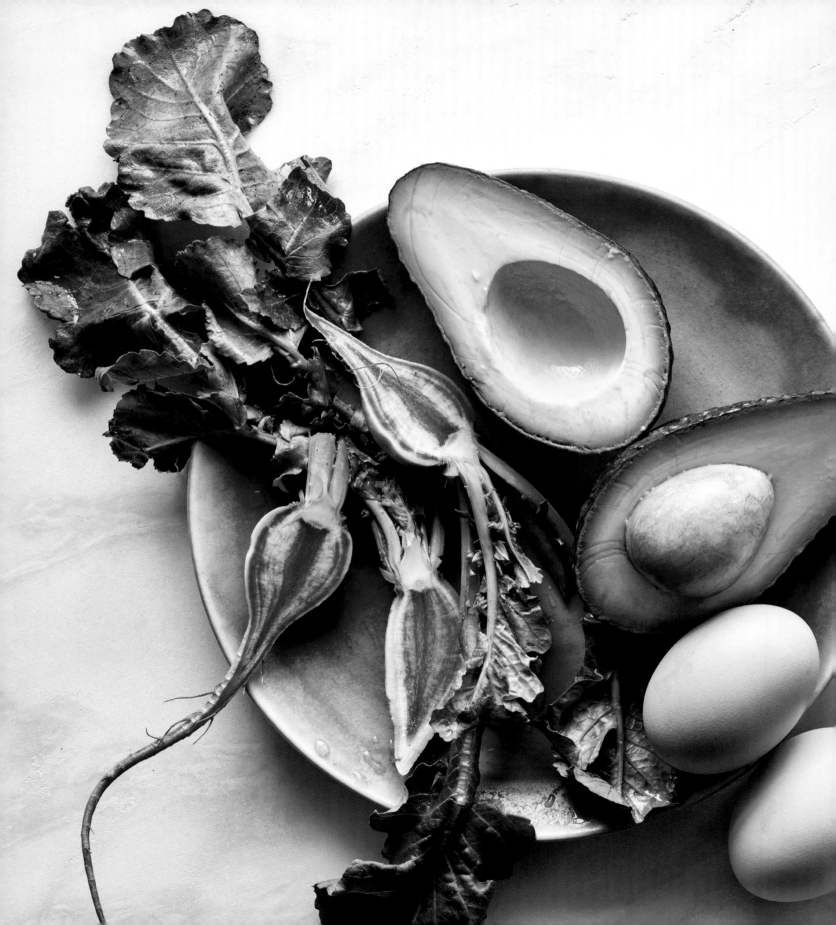

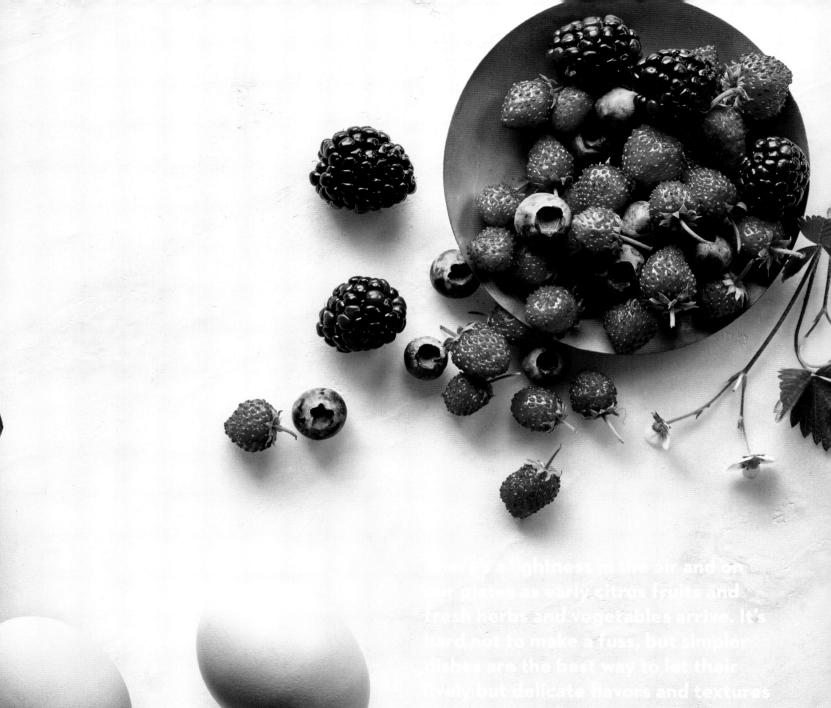

...ly a lightness in the air and on ...r plates as early citrus fruits and fresh herbs and vegetables arrive. It's hard not to make a fuss, but simpler dishes are the best way to let their lively but delicate flavors and textures take center stage.

# SPRING

It's wonderful that nature gives us so many cues to renew. Spring's first shoots add color back into our world, bring fresh flavors to our plates, and spark inspiration for growth. Thank you, spring!

In honor of the season of fresh starts, these recipes show just how easy and delicious it is to enjoy a SIBO-friendly, microbiome-balanced way of eating.

# perfect fried egg

**SERVES 1–2** | LF | V | GF

We love a perfectly cooked sunny-side up egg, with a runny yolk and a completely cooked white. Using a pan with a lid keeps the white tender yet fully cooked. Salted butter ensures a nicely seasoned egg. This recipe is for a single egg and is easily multiplied if you are cooking for more than one.

**INGREDIENTS**

1 teaspoon butter or olive oil

1 egg

Salt and freshly ground black pepper, to taste

**PREPARATION**

Over medium-low heat, add butter or olive oil to pan. If using olive oil, add a sprinkle of salt to the pan before adding egg. When butter is melted or oil is hot (about 1 minute) crack egg into pan and lightly sprinkle with salt and pepper. Cover with a lid and let steam for 3–4 minutes until white is just cooked through and yolk is still runny. If you prefer a more cooked yolk, continue cooking an additional 1–2 minutes.

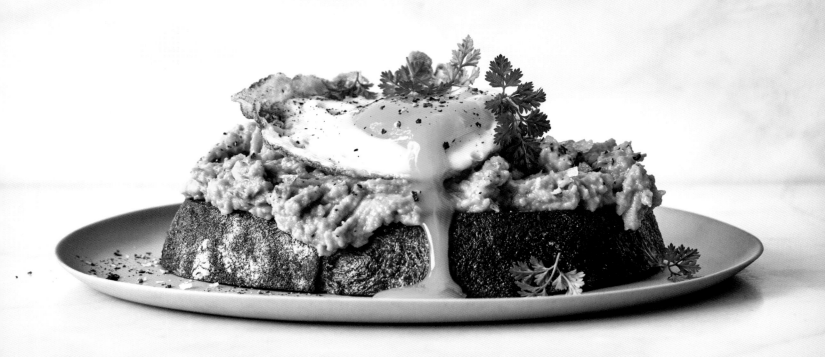

# new potato, leek, bacon & aged cheddar frittata

**SERVES 4-6** | GF

There is no disputing the ease and practicality of a frittata. This egg-based, one-pan wonder is a satisfying breakfast but can be served for any meal. If you need a bacon fix, this recipe has you covered. The leeks and cheese create a flavorful background.

## INGREDIENTS

4 pieces bacon, chopped

12 small fingerling, new potatoes, or other very small potatoes, thinly sliced

1 leek, thinly sliced

12 small fingerling, new potatoes, or other very small potatoes, thinly sliced

1 cup aged cheddar, grated

1 tablespoon thyme, chopped

### FOR EGGS:

12 eggs + 1 5.4 ounce can coconut cream + 1¼ teaspoon of salt blended in blender or with hand blender until frothy.

## PREPARATION

Preheat oven to 400°F (200°C).

Sauté bacon in cast iron pan over medium heat until slightly crispy. Remove from pan and set aside. Leave 2 tablespoons of fat in pan and discard remainder (or save for another time).

In batches, layer potatoes in a single layer, lightly salt, and fry for two minutes on each side. Set aside on plate when finished. After all the potatoes are cooked, sauté leeks with another pinch of salt for 10 minutes until soft and golden.

Layer one thin layer of potatoes on top of leeks. Top with half of the cheese, thyme, and bacon, then top with another layer of potatoes.

While pan is over low heat, pour in half the egg mixture, top with remaining cheese, then pour in remaining egg mixture. Cook on stovetop for 5–8 minutes until edges of frittata start to set.

Bake at 400°F (200°C) for 15 minutes until middle of frittata is almost completely set. It will continue to firm up over the next 10 minutes.

# protein pancakes *with* blueberry compote

**MAKES ABOUT 20 (4") PANCAKES
AND 1 ½ CUPS OF BLUEBERRY COMPOTE** | LF

Somewhere between a pancake and a crêpe, these thin vanilla-scented treats are a crowd pleaser. They reheat and freeze beautifully if you happen to have any leftovers. Add an extra ¼ cup almond milk to make extra-thin crêpes.

## INGREDIENTS

**PANCAKES:**

6 eggs

1 cup lactose-free cottage cheese

½ cup flour

¼ cup almond or lactose-free milk

¼ cup olive oil

2 tablespoons maple syrup

1 teaspoon vanilla extract

¼ teaspoon baking powder

¼ teaspoon salt

**COMPOTE:**

2 cups fresh or frozen blueberries

½ cup water

Juice from ¼ lemon

1 teaspoon maple syrup or to taste

## PREPARATION

Blend all pancake ingredients together in a blender for 1 minute until batter is smooth. Scrape blender with a spatula and blend for another 30 seconds. Heat a non-toxic, non-stick skillet or griddle over medium heat until hot. Use a ¼ cup measuring cup to pour batter into pan. Cook on each side until golden.

To make compote, combine all ingredients in a small sauce pot. Cook over medium-low heat for 20 minutes or until compote has thickened.

Serve pancakes alongside bowl of compote for people to spoon on top of their pancake stacks.

# Poppy's almond butter balls

**MAKES 25 (1") BALLS** | LF | V | GF

A fun project to do with kids, these are a simple grab-and-go snack filled with protein. Keep refrigerated so they maintain their shape.

**INGREDIENTS**

1½ cups almond or peanut butter

1 tablespoon honey

2 cups crispy rice cereal

**PREPARATION**

Thoroughly mix almond butter and honey together. Refrigerate for 30 minutes. Place crispy rice cereal in a small bowl. With your hands, roll teaspoon-sized scoops of almond butter into balls and roll in cereal. Roll again in your hands to make sure cereal sticks to outside of balls. After balls are made, place in an airtight container and refrigerate for at least 30 minutes before eating.

# sweet cashew cream *with* mixed berries

**MAKES 1 CUP** | LF | V | GF

This can be served on its own as a pudding-like dessert. It also makes a fantastic whipped cream substitute topping for cakes, pies, and sundaes.

**INGREDIENTS**

**FOR CASHEW CREAM:**

1½ cup cashew, soaked 1 hour in water and drained

¼ cup water + more if needed to make creamy

1 teaspoon vanilla extract

1 teaspoon maple syrup

¼ teaspoon salt

Zest from 1 lemon

1 teaspoon lemon juice

**GARNISH WITH:**

1 pint mixed berries

Dark chocolate, shaved

Mint leaves

**PREPARATION**

Combine all cashew cream ingredients in a blender and blend until smooth and creamy.

Serve berries topped with cashew cream, shaved chocolate, and a mint leaf garnish.

# pecan sweet potato bars

**MAKES ONE 8 × 12" SHEET PAN** | LF | V | GF

Slightly sweet and full of protein, these make a great grab-and-go snack or an after-dinner sweet.

## INGREDIENTS

### CRUST:

2½ cups toasted pecans

4 tablespoons melted coconut oil

1 teaspoon maple syrup

⅛ teaspoon salt

### FILLING:

1½ cups baked + pureed sweet potatoes
(about 3 medium sweet potatoes)

1 cup lactose-free whey protein isolate

1 cup almond meal

1 teaspoon cinnamon

Maple syrup, to taste

### TOPPING:

1 cup chopped pecans

2 tablespoons maple syrup

Large pinch salt

## PREPARATION

Preheat oven to 325°F (165°C).

For crust, pulse first four ingredients in a food processor until you have a coarse, crumbly mixture that resembles coarse sand. Press evenly into the bottom of an 8 × 12" sheet pan. To make filling, mix sweet potatoes, whey protein, almond meal, cinnamon, and sweeten to taste with maple syrup. Spread filling over crust and bake at 325°F (165°C) for 15 minutes, rotating half-way through. While bars are baking, toss chopped pecans with maple syrup and salt in a sauté pan and toast over medium heat until sticky (about 3–5 minutes), then spread evenly over top of finished bars. Refrigerate until completely cooled and cut into squares.

*Exercise is an important part of any healthy lifestyle, but especially for anyone striving for microbiome balance. Evidence suggests that exercise can directly and beneficially alter the composition of your gut microbiome. These post-workout snacks pack all a body needs to properly refuel and repair. Ideally eat within an hour of exercise, while still maintaining the four-hour gut-cleansing windows between meals and snacks.*

## A FEW NUTRITIONAL HIGHLIGHTS

**SWEET POTATOES:** especially rich in potassium, an important electrolyte that is lost through sweat

**ALMONDS + RICE:** protein, carbohydrates, and calories that promote muscle recovery, restore lost glycogen stores, and maintain healthy blood sugar levels

**CASHEWS:** an excellent source of plant-based protein, which aids in muscle recovery and growth

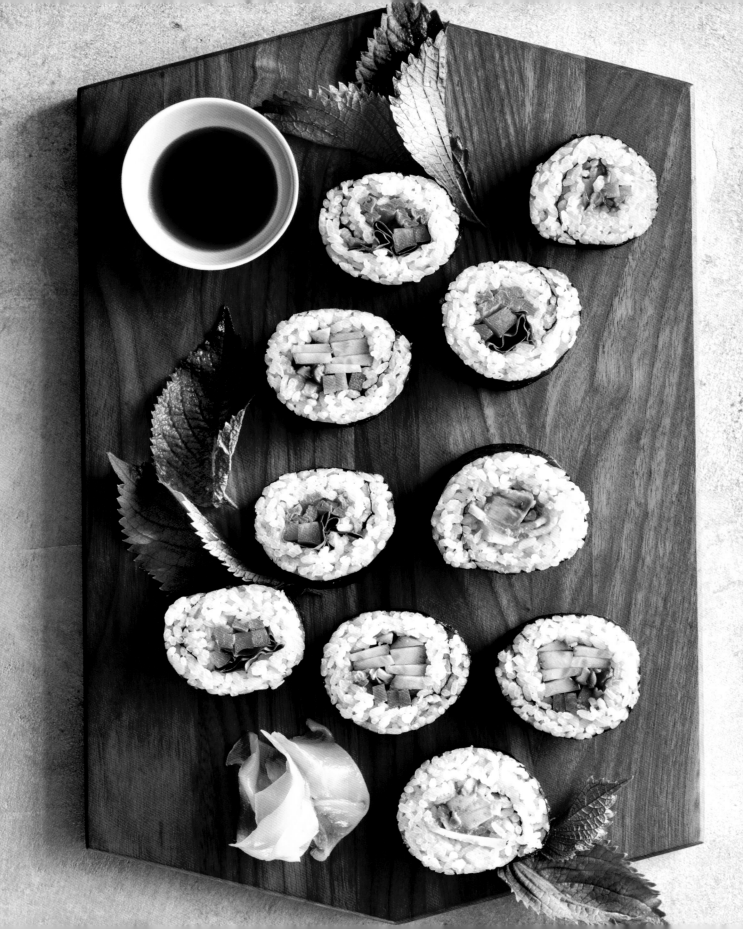

# veggie sushi rolls

**MAKES 6 (8-PIECE) ROLLS** | LF | V | GF

Sushi is easier to make than you think and makes for a fun roll-your-own sushi dinner party. You don't need a bamboo mat—a clean kitchen towel does the trick. Prep all the fillings, lay out on plates, and let people create their own combinations.

## INGREDIENTS

2½ cups sushi rice

2½ cups water

2 tablespoons rice vinegar, mixed with:
    1 tablespoon sugar
    1 tablespoon salt

1 package nori sheets

High-quality wasabi powder

Pickled ginger

### IDEAS FOR FILLINGS:

English cucumber, peeled and sliced into long ¼" matchsticks, sprinkled with salt

Handful shiitake mushrooms, sliced and sautéed with salt and coconut aminos

Sweet potato, peeled, sliced into long ¼" matchsticks and tossed in olive oil, salted and roasted

Ripe avocado, sliced thinly and sprinkled with salt and lemon juice

Carrots, julienned or grated

Mango, sliced into long ¼" matchsticks

Toasted macadamia nuts, chopped

Fresh ginger, finely grated

Basil, cut in chiffonade

Mint, cut in chiffonade

Shizo leaf, cut in chiffonade

## PREPARATION

Rinse rice in strainer until water runs clear. Put in saucepan (with tight-fitting lid), add water and bring to boil, uncovered. Turn down heat, cover, and cook for 15 minutes. Then turn off heat and let sit, covered, for 10 minutes before transferring to large mixing bowl (or cook according to rice package). Pour rice vinegar mixture over top of rice and toss with fork or large wooden spoon. Let rice come to room temperature before assembling sushi.

To assemble, place one sheet of nori on a clean kitchen towel. Dip hands in small bowl of water and use wet fingers to press sushi rice onto nori in a ¼" layer, leaving 1" of space at the furthest edge of nori. Place a long line of desired fillings 1" from closest edge of rice covered nori. Wet open edge of nori with water and use dish towel to tightly roll into a long log. Use a sharp knife to cut each roll into 8 pieces. Serve with pickled ginger, coconut aminos, and wasabi for dipping.

# carrot romesco

**MAKES 1 CUP** | LF | V | GF

Typically made with peppers, this carrot-based romesco is a nutritious, versatile spread that can be used as a dip with crackers or crostini, as a topping for baked fish, or tossed with pasta for a quick weeknight dinner. It also makes a great vegan ravioli filling.

**INGREDIENTS**

4 carrots cut into large chunks

5 cloves garlic, peeled

½ cup almonds

Small handful of parsley

Juice and zest of ½ lemon

¼–½ teaspoons smoked paprika (season to preferred smokiness)

2 tablespoons water

3 tablespoons olive oil

Salt, to taste

**PREPARATION**

Preheat oven to 450°F (230°C)

On a parchment-lined sheet pan, toss carrots with 1 tablespoon olive oil and a large pinch of salt. Roast for 15 minutes. Add garlic to sheet pan and roast for another 15 minutes. Add almonds to sheet pan and roast for final 10 minutes. (For total of 40 minutes.)

Let cool and add carrots, almonds, and garlic to food processor along with handful of parsley, lemon juice and zest, smoked paprika, water, and remaining olive oil. Pulse until almonds are in small bits and carrots are creamy. Add an additional tablespoon of water and oil and blend further if you want a creamier consistency.

Season to taste with lemon and salt.

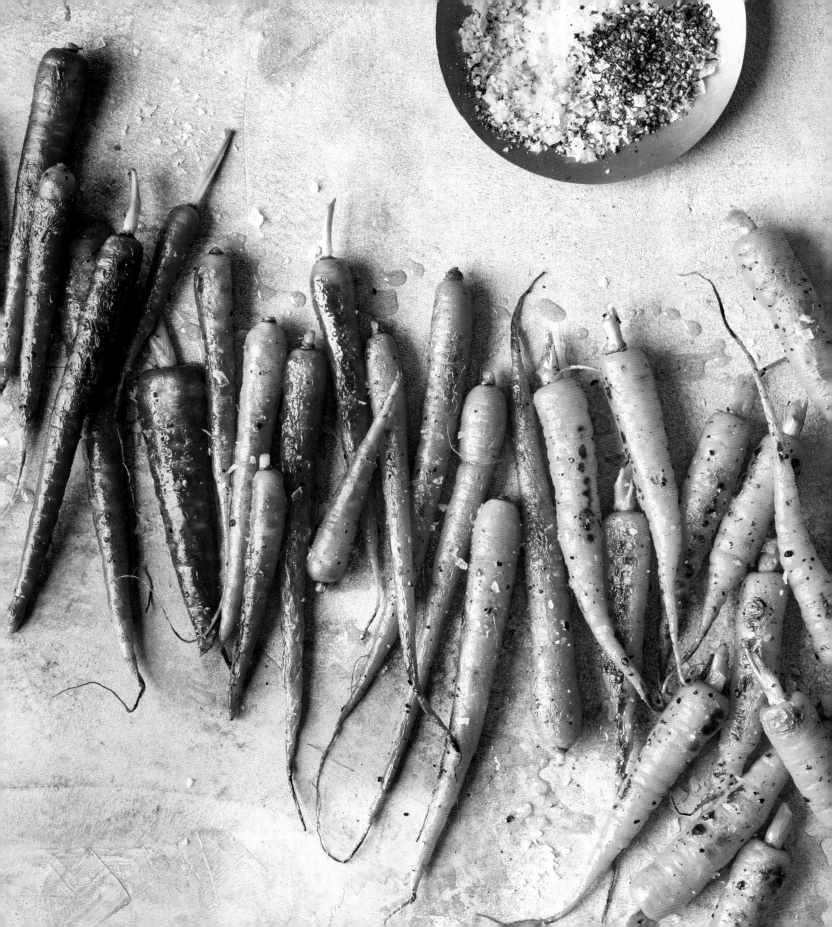

# tzatziki

**MAKES 2 CUPS** | LF | V | GF

This gets better after it sits for a few hours in the refrigerator, so it's a great recipe to make in advance.

---

### INGREDIENTS

½ recipe Cashew Sour Cream (p. 124)

**WITH:**

2 tablespoons of olive oil while blending

Additional juice and zest of 1 lemon

1 garlic clove, grated on microplane

1½ cups cucumber, grated,
and 1 tablespoon reserved for garnish

5 stems mint, leaves picked
and finely chopped

1 tablespoon garlic olive oil

Salt and freshly ground black pepper, to taste

### PREPARATION

Make Cashew Sour Cream (p. 124) and while blending add olive oil, lemon juice, garlic, lemon zest, and salt.

Scrape cream into medium mixing bowl and stir in cucumber and mint. Add water as needed to make a creamy sauce. Season to taste with salt and pepper. Top with garlic olive oil and a little grated cucumber.

# guacamole

**MAKES 2 ½ CUPS** | LF | V | GF

There are so many dressed-up versions of guacamole, but little more is needed than perfectly ripe avocados smashed with a few squeezes of lime juice, some fresh cilantro, a little onion for crunch, and a touch of spice. Simplicity at its finest. It's delicious with crispy tortilla chips, or spread on a warm corn tortilla and topped with an over-easy egg for breakfast.

---

### INGREDIENTS

6 ripe avocados, mashed with fork

½ medium red onion, minced

½ bunch cilantro leaves, minced

Juice of 2–3 limes, to taste

Zest of 1 lime

1 teaspoon jalapeño, minced
(or dried cayenne powder, to taste)

Salt and freshly ground black pepper, to taste

### PREPARATION

Combine mashed avocado, red onion, cilantro, lime juice, and zest, and jalapeños (or cayenne powder). Season with salt, pepper, and lime juice.

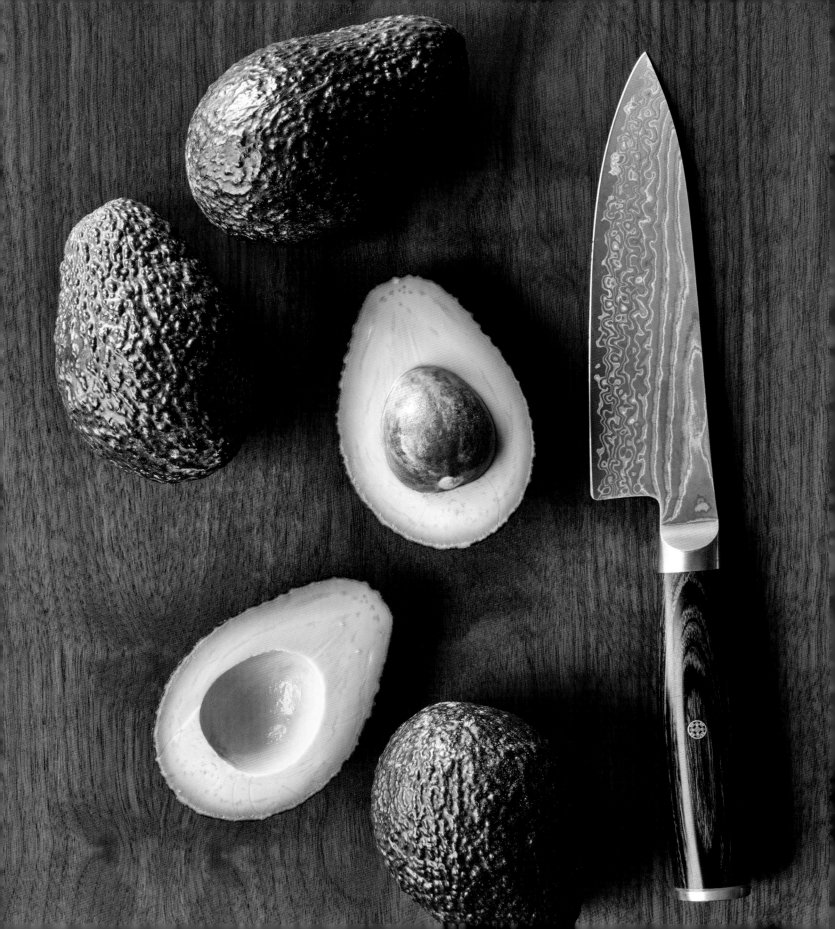

# herb salad

**MAKES 1 PINT** | LF | V | GF

More of a condiment than a salad, herb salad is like a deconstructed salsa verde that can add a fresh element to grilled fish, frittatas, grilled meats or vegetables, roasted potatoes, or even on top of a pizza. I'll add a few shavings of fresh grated horseradish if I'm using it as a topping for red meat.

### INGREDIENTS

Handful parsley, picked into individual leaves

1 bunch chives, cut into 1" sticks

4 sprigs tarragon, picked into individual leaves

½ bunch chervil or cilantro sprouts, picked (optional)

Zest of 1 lemon

Olive oil

Lemon juice

Crunchy salt

### PREPARATION

When ready to serve, gently toss all herbs with a very light dressing of olive oil and a light squeeze of lemon.

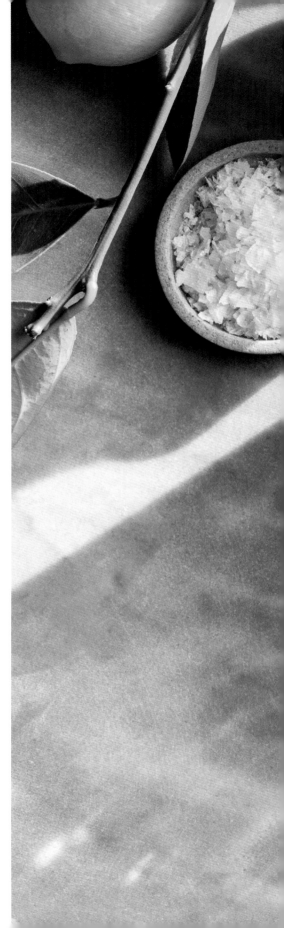

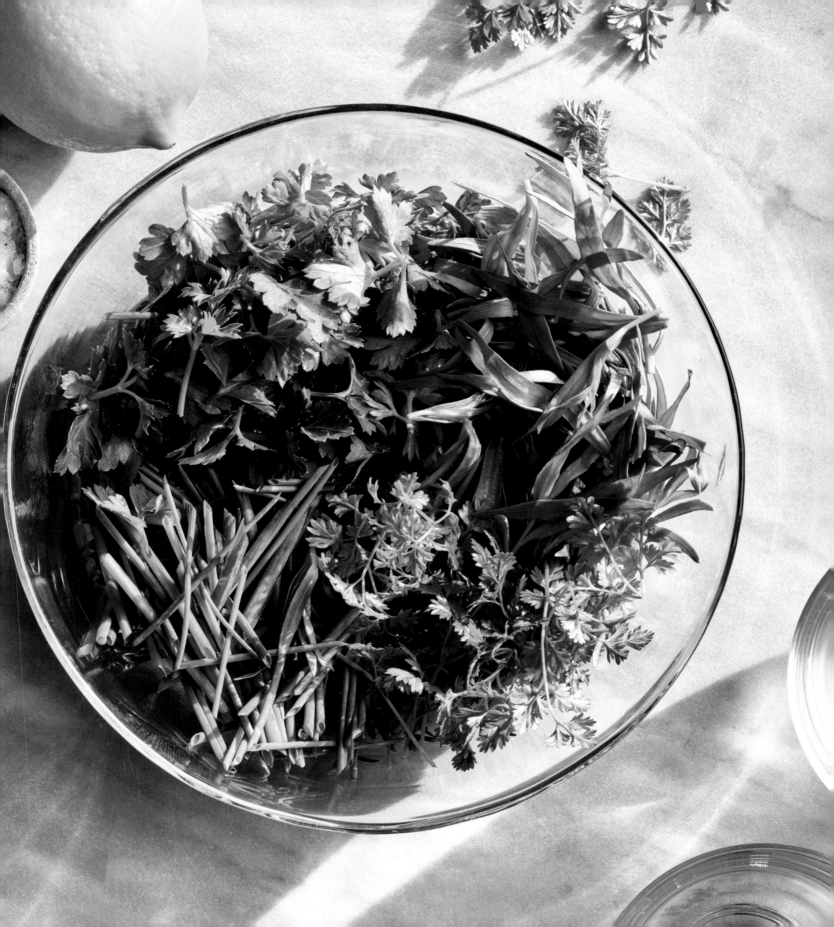

# insalata tricolore

**SERVES 6 (as a side dish)** | LF | V | GF

A classic Italian salad that gets its name from the three colors of the Italian flag. The combination of bitter lettuces and a bright lemon citronette is a refreshing start to a meal.

**INGREDIENTS**

3 endives, outside layer peeled

1 head radicchio, outside layer peeled

4 ounces arugula, washed

2 tablespoons Lemon Citronette (p. 25)

Parmesan cheese, shaved with a vegetable peeler

Salt and freshly ground pepper, to taste

**PREPARATION**

Keep all the lettuces separate in three bowls. Slice endive into 1" pieces and place in first bowl. Cut head of radicchio in half and remove the hard white core. Slice very thinly into long strips and place in second bowl. Place arugula in third bowl. Add ⅓ of the citronette to each bowl with a small pinch of salt and ground black pepper, mix until evenly coated. Plate each lettuce in the shape of the Italian flag; arugula, endive, and radicchio in that order. Top with shaved Parmesan cheese.

# zucchini & parmesan salad

**SERVES 6-8** | LF | V | GF

An invigorating, elegant use of summer's abundance of zucchini.

**INGREDIENTS**

3 zucchini + 3 carrots, peeled into long ribbons with a vegetable peeler

6 radishes, thinly sliced

1 bunch mint, chiffonaded

½ cup Parmesan cheese, shaved into strips with vegetable peeler

1 recipe Dijon Vinaigrette (p. 25), using about 2 tablespoons for this recipe

**PREPARATION**

For the dressing, place shallots and vinegar in a small jar and marinate until shallots turn bright pink—about 15 minutes. Add remaining ingredients, screw lid on jar, and shake until well combined.

Combine carrots, zucchini, radishes, and mint in a large bowl. Toss vegetables with a light coat of dressing. Season to taste with salt and ground pepper. Top with Parmesan cheese shavings and shallots.

# dijon vinaigrette

**MAKES ½ CUP** | LF | V | GF

I always make my vinaigrettes in a container with a tightly fitting lid, like a mason jar, so I can just add all the ingredients together and give it a good shake. This is a classic, versatile vinaigrette, equally good on leafy greens, steamed vegetables, or used to marinate chicken before roasting. Add honey if you prefer a little sweetness to your dressings.

## INGREDIENTS

½ shallot, thinly sliced

2½ tablespoons red wine vinegar

¼ cup olive oil

1½ tablespoon Dijon mustard

1 tablespoon tarragon, chopped

1 tablespoon parsley, chopped

Zest of 1 lemon

1 teaspoon honey (optional)

## PREPARATION

Let shallot marinate in red vinegar for a few minutes before adding additional ingredients. Add all ingredients to jar and shake.

# lemon citronette

**MAKES ½ CUP** | LF | V | GF

A classic lemon dressing that is delicious on bitter greens with radishes. I sometimes forget how refreshingly simple a dressing can be. This one is a reminder that it doesn't have to be complicated to be good.

## INGREDIENTS

Juice and zest of 1 lemon

⅓ cup olive oil

½ shallot, diced

2 pinches salt

## PREPARATION

Add all ingredients to jar and shake.

# green bean potato salad

**SERVES 6-8** | LF | V | GF

A lighter version of potato salad and great for summer picnics. Leftovers can easily transform into a Niçoise salad. For a full lunchtime meal, add a handful of olives, a boiled egg, and tuna.

### INGREDIENTS

6 Yukon Gold potatoes, scrubbed

$\frac{1}{2}$ pound green beans, ends trimmed and cut into 2" pieces

2 tablespoons whole grain or Dijon mustard

2 tablespoons each, chives and tarragon, chopped

Zest of 1 lemon

$\frac{1}{2}$ shallot, thinly sliced and macerated in 1 tablespoon red wine vinegar

2 tablespoons olive oil

Salt and freshly ground black pepper, to taste

### PREPARATION

Place whole, cleaned potatoes in a saucepan of cold water. Bring to a simmer and cook for 35–45 minutes or until a knife can easily go through potatoes. Steam green beans until tender, then cool in an ice bath. When potatoes are cooked, cut into 1" chunks. Mix mustard, herbs, lemon zest, vinegar and shallot, and oil together to make dressing. Season to taste and gently toss potatoes, green beans, and dressing together.

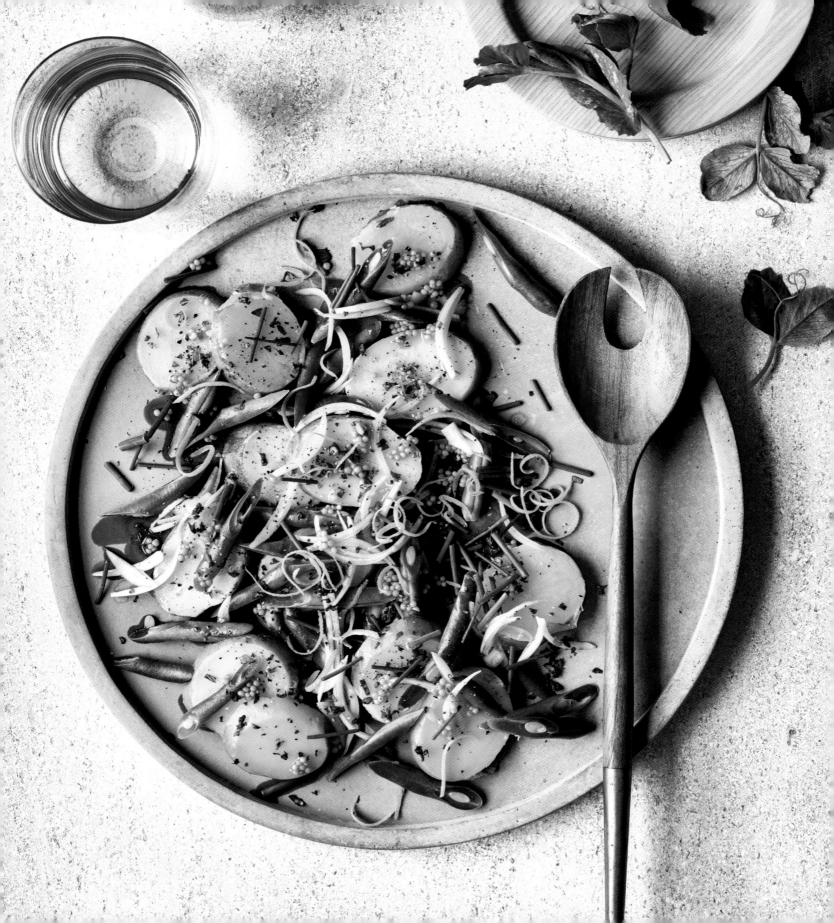

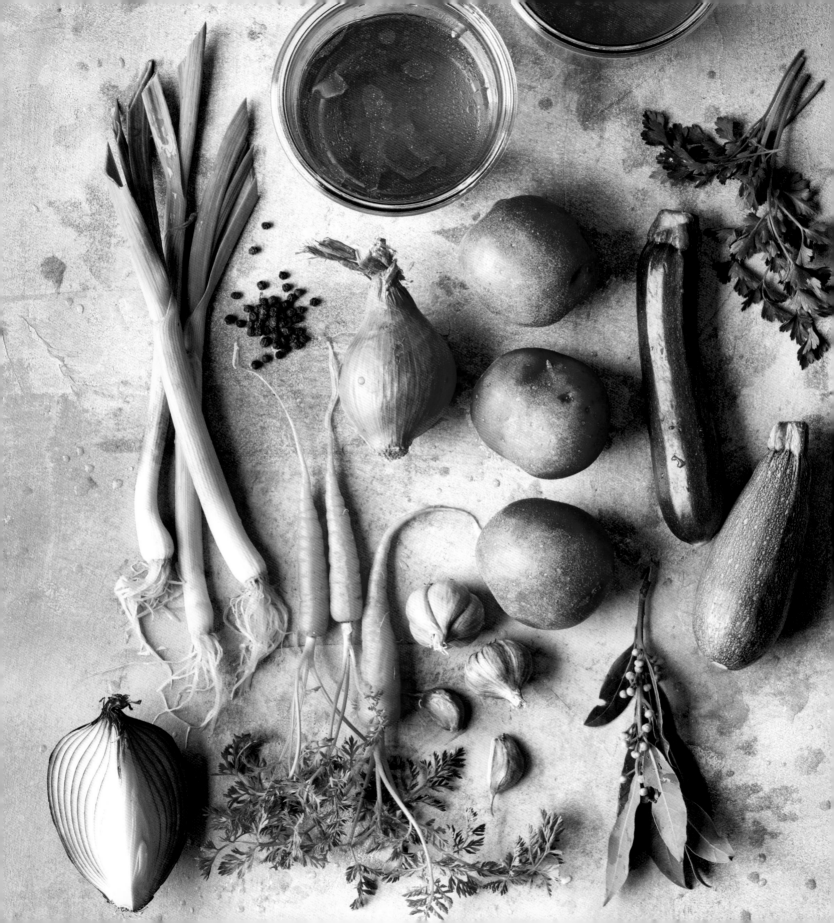

# mineral-rich vegetable broth

**MAKES ABOUT 4 QUARTS** | LF | V | GF

This is a basic broth that can be used in a variety of recipes. It's good on its own when recovering from colds or when you are feeling under the weather. I drink it by the mugful when I am not feeling well. Since the vegetables are roasted, it has a deep flavor and can substitute for chicken broth if you are vegetarian.

## INGREDIENTS

4 stalks celery

4 carrots

1 leek (you can use another onion if leeks are not readily available)

1 onion

1 large sweet potato or 2 small

2 potatoes (can be any kind)

5 cloves garlic

2 zucchini

Olive oil

1 tablespoon vinegar (wine vinegar)

4–5 quarts water (just enough to cover vegetables by a couple of inches)

5 stems thyme

¼ bunch parsley (omit for pregnant women and women who are breastfeeding)

Salt and freshly ground black pepper, to taste

\* I have tried using the whole leek because it seems like a shame to throw so much of it away, but it ends up making a bitter stock.

\* Here's a space-saving tip: after straining, return liquid to the pot and reduce by half. This will make a more concentrated broth, taking up less space in the refrigerator or freezer.

## PREPARATION

Preheat oven to 450°F (230°C). Wash herbs and vegetables. Cut tops and ends off of all vegetables. For leeks, leave about 2" of greens.\* Cut celery, carrots, leeks, and onions into large chunks (about 1"). Submerge leeks in a large bowl of water, swish around to loosen dirt. Change water a couple of times until there is no grit in bottom of bowl. Use a salad spinner or air-dry.

Place onion (leave skin on if organic), and all other vegetables, except for zucchini, on a parchment-lined baking sheet. Add a couple of big splashes of olive oil (about 2–3 tablespoons), 1 teaspoon of salt, and about 15 grinds of pepper. Mix around until coated. Roast for about 35 minutes until soft and caramelized. You can skip this step and just brown vegetables in the pot before adding water. However, I find if I have the time, roasting creates a richer, more complex stock. And it makes the house smell good!

Chop zucchini into large, rough chunks. Put in stockpot. Add roasted vegetables and vinegar, then cover with **cold** water. Starting a vegetable stock with cold water helps extract the nutrients that dissolve at different temperatures. It keeps the vegetables in whole chunks for a little longer, making straining easier. Bring to a low simmer (**not** boiling) and as foam rises to the surface, skim off. Let simmer for 2 hours. Add herbs for last half hour of simmering. From here you can season to taste with salt and ground pepper. I like to leave it under-seasoned so it's a versatile, neutral addition to other recipes.

Strain and ladle into large jars to freeze (will keep for several months) or keep in refrigerator for up to 4 days. Because this doesn't have the fats and protein of a meat-based broth, it won't last long in the fridge.

# pesto genovese

**MAKES 1 CUP** | LF | V | GF

Like salsa verde, this recipe turns into something extra special when you chop the ingredients by hand. You'll want to make sure your knife is super sharp so the basil can be finely chopped without bruising. It all comes together quickly and is great on top of baked salmon, stirred into a rustic vegetable soup, or with your favorite noodles with herbed breadcrumb topping.

### INGREDIENTS

Handful of grated Parmesan or Romano cheese

3 cloves garlic, grated (optional)

¼ cup pine nuts, lightly toasted

1 bunch basil, washed and stems picked off

3 tablespoons olive oil or garlic-infused olive oil if not using raw garlic

Couple pinches of salt

### PREPARATION

Pile cheese, garlic (if using), and pine nuts in the middle of a large cutting board and place basil on top. Going from left to right, roughly chop all of the ingredients together. When you get to the right side, scoop all ingredients back into a pile and chop again. Repeat this process about 10–15 times until everything is chopped into a very rough paste. Scoop all ingredients into a bowl and top with olive oil. Stir and season to taste.

# puttanesca

**MAKES 3 ½ CUPS** | LF | GF

Puttanesca is a flavorful last-minute pasta sauce. Anchovies add a richness to this sauce; cooking them over low heat ensures they don't get too fishy.

### INGREDIENTS

1 large can diced tomatoes or 3 cups Simple Summertime Tomato Sauce (p. 79)

½ cup dry white wine

3 garlic cloves, diced

2 tablespoons capers, diced

4 anchovy fillets, chopped

¾ cup Kalamata olives, chopped

1 teaspoon chili flakes

### PREPARATION

Cook tomatoes in saucepan with wine for 30 minutes. While tomatoes are simmering, sauté garlic, capers, anchovies, chili flakes, and olives over low heat until garlic is fragrant and lightly toasted. Stir into tomatoes and let cook for 15 minutes.

# traditional red sauce

**MAKES 1 QUART** | LF | V | GF

Here's a basic but tasty pasta sauce. We sometimes double or triple the recipe and freeze leftovers to make for a quick weeknight pasta dinner.

## INGREDIENTS

1 onion, diced

2 celery ribs, diced

2 carrots, diced

1 large can organic diced tomatoes or 4 cups of Simple Summertime Tomato Sauce (p. 79)

½ cup dry red or white wine

2 cloves garlic, diced

Pinch dried red chili flakes (optional)

1 tablespoon fresh oregano, minced

10 fresh basil leaves, chiffonaded

Salt and freshly ground black pepper, to taste

Olive oil

## PREPARATION

In a medium saucepan, sauté onion, celery, and carrots with a generous pour of olive oil over medium heat. Cook for 10 minutes until all are lightly golden and fragrant. Add tomatoes, wine, and a couple pinches of salt. Continue to cook over medium heat for 10 minutes until alcohol aroma has cooked out. Lower heat, add one can of water to sauce and cook for 1 hour or until sauce has thickened. As sauce is cooking, sauté garlic in a small frying pan with a small amount of olive oil until fragrant but not brown. Add chili flakes to garlic if using. When sauce is done simmering add garlic and chili flake mixture, season to taste with salt and pepper. Add herbs before tossing with your favorite pasta or pasta substitute.

*Remember, digestion begins in the mouth; take time to chew, taste, and enjoy. Your microbiome will thank you.*

# sautéed zucchini *with* red onions *&* lime

**MAKES 1 ½ QUARTS** | LF | V | GF

Zucchini has a mild flavor and most people think it demands layers and layers of flavors but in actuality, it can sing on its own with the addition of just a few simple ingredients. Prepare to be surprised!

## INGREDIENTS

1 zucchini + 2 summer squash cut into quarters lengthwise and sliced into quarter moons ¼" thick

2 garlic cloves, sliced thinly

1 teaspoon coriander

Zest and juice from 1 lime

2 tablespoons olive oil

1 small red onion, sliced thinly

2 pinches sea salt

Salt and freshly ground black pepper, to taste

## PREPARATION

In a very large sauté pan or cast iron skillet, heat olive oil. Add onion with a pinch of salt and sauté 4 minutes over medium heat. Add the zucchini, squash, garlic, coriander, and two large pinches sea salt. Cook, stirring, about 8–12 minutes, until just tender. Stir in lime zest, juice, and black pepper. Adjust seasoning to taste.

# AN ODE TO ZUCCHINI

*Don't let its ubiquity fool you into thinking that this familiar vegetable isn't special. Packed with nutrition, versatile, and easy to digest, zucchini holds a special place in our hearts and on our plates. Here's also why it's one of the most SIBO-friendly vegetables around:*

---

- Zucchini has a 94% water content, making it hydrating and easy on the digestive system.

- Zucchini has a high fiber component, encourages gut motility, and helps to cleanse the digestive tract.

- It's lower in many of the fermentable carbohydrates that can cause problems for those with digestive issues.

- Beyond its nutritional benefits, zucchini's mild flavor lets it pair well with almost any dish, from zesty lemon-based fish dishes to savory roasted meats.

- Zucchini is rich in minerals and vitamins including: potassium, phosphorus, magnesium, calcium, sodium, zinc, iron, vitamins A, B6 and riboflavin, C, E, and K.

- Slice it, spiral it, use it in place of pasta, or add to your scrambled eggs for a bit of texture and fiber; it's the vegetable of a thousand faces.

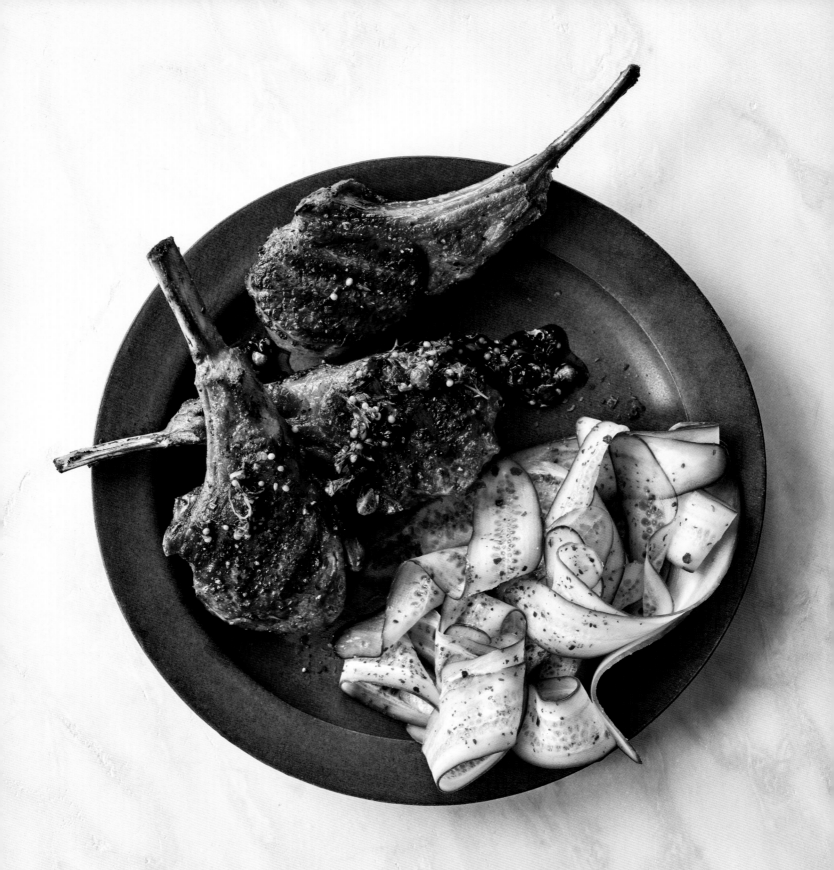

# rosemary & olive oil lamb chops

**MAKES 8 SERVINGS** | LF | GF

Lemony sumac balances the gaminess of the lamb. Great with salsa verde or herb salad, these can be a quick weeknight dinner or dinner party fare. Make sure to remove any garlic before grilling as it will burn. As for the rosemary, enjoy crispy bits in each bite, but if you would like something more refined, remove the rosemary before grilling.

## INGREDIENTS

18–24 lamb chops (depending on size)

½ cup rosemary, roughly chopped (about 3 large sprigs)

8 garlic cloves, crushed and left mostly whole

1½ tablespoons sumac (save ½ tablespoon for finishing)

3 tablespoons olive oil

1 tablespoon salt + crunchy salt to finish

Freshly ground black pepper

## PREPARATION

Lay chops out on sheet pan. Season both sides of chops with salt and a couple grinds of black pepper per chop. Combine rosemary, garlic, sumac, and olive oil to make a loose paste, then cover both sides of chops with mixture. Cover and let rest in refrigerator for 3 hours. Remove from refrigerator 1 hour before cooking. Remove garlic pieces from chops and heat a large pan over high heat—I prefer a well-used cast iron pan, but a large stainless steel sauté pan will work, too. When pan is hot enough to sizzle, cook chops for 2–3 minutes on each side, including the thin sides: so 4 sides total. For smaller chops, cook for 2 minutes on each side, for larger chops cook for 3 minutes one each side.

Remove from heat and sprinkle with remaining sumac, crunchy salt, and a grind of pepper for each chop.

You can also cook these on the grill for 5 minutes on each side.

# lemongrass chicken lettuce wraps

**MAKES 12–18 WRAPS** | LF | GF

These are great served with carrot jicama slaw or pickled carrots. I often serve these family-style with toppings and lettuce in little bowls so everyone can assemble their own wraps.

## INGREDIENTS

10 chicken thighs

**MARINADE:**

2 stalks lemongrass
or ¼ cup dried lemongrass

Large handful kaffir lime leaves
or zest of 3 limes

1 tablespoon fish sauce or coconut aminos

1 shallot chopped into rough pieces

¼ cup olive oil

1 tablespoon Sriracha or chili paste

**TO SERVE:**

1 head butter lettuce

1 cup cherry tomatoes, quartered

3 green onions, thinly sliced

Cucumbers, sliced and tossed with
rice vinegar and a pinch of sugar

Carrot and jicama slaw or pickled carrots

Lime slices

## PREPARATION

Marinate chicken thighs for a minimum of
2 hours or overnight.

Wipe excess marinade off chicken and cook in
large, well-oiled skillet for 4 minutes on each
side or until thighs are cooked through. Let
cooked chicken rest for 5 minutes and slice thinly.
Chicken can also be grilled over medium-high
heat until cooked through.

To assemble, place a few slices of chicken on
lettuce and top with vegetables and slaw.

# chicken kebabs

**MAKES ABOUT 12 SKEWERS** | LF | GF

This colorful weeknight dinner can be seasoned in different ways depending on what marinade you use. The lemon and herb marinade goes well with Greek or Italian menus, while the garlic and curry marinade is fantastic with peanut sauce and an Asian inspired salad. Loosely stack your meat and vegetables on skewers to ensure they cook evenly. Soaking your onions in salt water reduces their bite.

## INGREDIENTS

### FOR SKEWERS:

10 boneless and skinless chicken thighs, cut into 1 × 2" strips

3 bell peppers (I like to use 1 each of red, green, and yellow) cut into 1" cubes

1 red onion, cut into 1" cubes, soaked in salt water for 30 minutes before marinating

### CURRY MARINADE:

½ cup coconut aminos

3 tablespoons rice vinegar

2 tablespoons maple syrup or brown sugar

1½ teaspoons mild curry powder

3 garlic cloves, grated

1 teaspoon salt

### LEMON AND HERB MARINADE:

½ cup olive oil

Juice and zest from 3 lemons

2 tablespoons thyme, chopped

2 tablespoon oregano, chopped

2 tablespoons Dijon mustard

3 garlic cloves, grated

2 teaspoons salt

Freshly ground black pepper, to taste

## PREPARATION

Assemble kebabs, alternating chicken and vegetables on skewers (folding chicken strips in half, if necessary). Place kebabs in large baking dish and pour marinade over top. Let marinate for 3 hours minimum, rotating to make sure all kebabs are evenly coated in marinade.

After kebabs have marinated, preheat oven to 350°F (180°C). Remove excesss marinade and bake on a large parchment-lined sheet pan for 30–45 minutes until chicken is cooked through. Turn oven to broil and broil for 1–2 minutes on each side until vegetables are slightly charred around edges.

The kebabs can also be grilled over medium heat. If grilling, soak skewers in water for 1 hour before assembling kebabs.

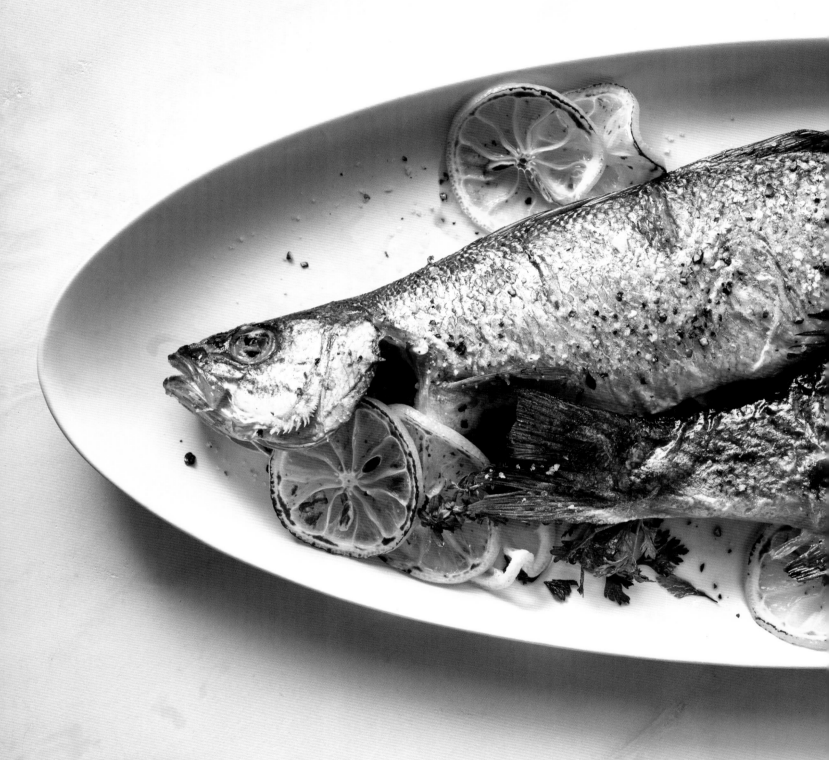

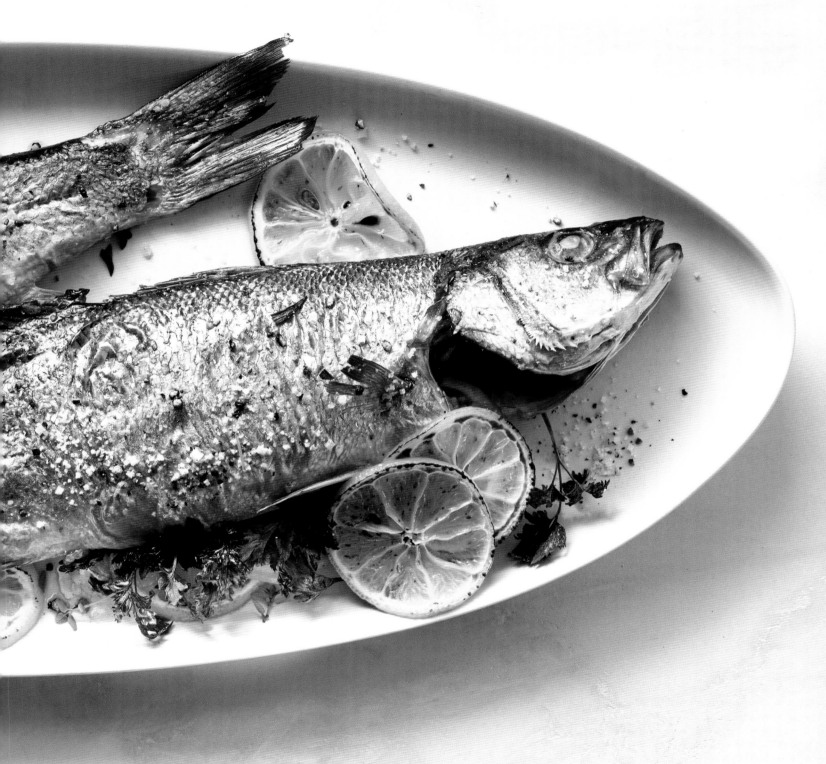

Branzino Stuffed with Herbs and Lemon / *recipe on following page*

# branzino stuffed *with* herbs *&* lemon

**SERVES 6–8** | LF | GF

This is a simple and beautiful way to cook a freshly caught fish. I always ask my fishmonger what the freshest fish of the day is, so any similarly sized fish will work in this recipe—wild caught rainbow trout and striped bass are favorite options.

## INGREDIENTS

4 whole branzino (1 –1 ¼ pounds), each scaled and gutted

Sea salt

2 lemons, sliced in ¼" rounds, seeds removed

1 bunch thyme

1 bunch parsley

Extra virgin olive oil

## PREPARATION

Preheat oven to 450°F (230°C). Line a large baking sheet with parchment paper.

Season each branzino with salt, on skin and inside the cavity of the fish. Place three lemon slices, a few sprigs of thyme, and a few sprigs of parsley inside of each branzino. Lightly oil the skin of the fish.

Bake for 15–18 minutes until fish is almost cooked through. Turn oven to broil and broil for 5 minutes until top of fish is bronzed and bubbly.

# grilled tuna *with* orange, grapefruit & olive oil

**MAKES 6 FILLETS** | LF | GF

Light and bright, and very quick to make, this is great on top of a watercress or arugula salad, or rice. Add leftovers to the Green Bean Potato Salad (p. 26) to create a Niçoise salad.

## INGREDIENTS

6 tuna steaks, 1" thick (about 1¾–2 pounds)

3 oranges, rinds cut off, cut into segments

3 grapefruit, rinds cut off, cut into segments

2 tablespoons olive oil

Coconut aminos

Coarse salt and freshly ground black pepper, to taste

## PREPARATION

Lightly season both sides of steaks with salt and pepper and rub with a tablespoon of olive oil. Heat a grill pan over medium-high heat for 1 minute until hot, then add steaks to pan. Cook fish for 3 minutes on each side (1½–2 minutes if you prefer your tuna rare). Toss citrus with olive oil and a sprinkle of coarse salt and a few grinds of pepper. Top each filet with a drizzle of coconut aminos and a large spoonful of citrus.

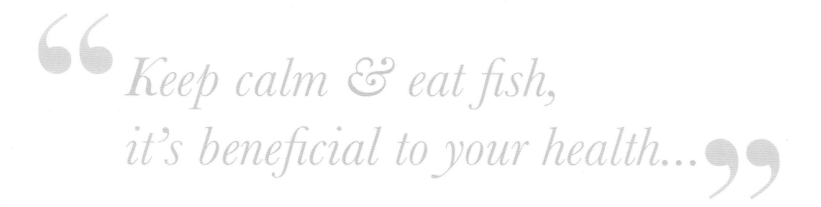

"*Keep calm & eat fish, it's beneficial to your health...*"

# chewy meringues & lemon curd

**SERVES 6 (with 6 meringues leftover to eat the next day)** | LF | V | GF

The classic solution to using both the whites and yolks of eggs is a custard pie topped with meringue. This deconstructed crustless version gives you a sweet meringue that is crispy outside with a chewy, marshmallow interior, all balanced by tart lemon curd. I actually like this curd made with ghee better than the traditional recipes that use butter. A little lighter and more fresh tasting—letting the lemon shine through.

## INGREDIENTS

**MERINGUE
(MAKES ABOUT A DOZEN MERINGUES):**

½ cup room temperature whites
(from about 3 large eggs)

1 cup sugar

¼ teaspoon cream of tartar

**LEMON CURD:**

3 egg yolks

¼ cup caster sugar

Zest of 2 lemons

Juice of 2–3 lemons (¼ cup)

4 tablespoons ghee

## PREPARATION

Preheat oven to 300°F (150°C) and line one 18 × 26" baking sheet with parchment paper.

Wash all bowls and mixing equipment in hot soapy water, dry thoroughly, and wipe with vinegar on a paper towel.

Separate yolks and whites being careful not to get any yolks into the whites. If you are wary of your separating skills you can separate them individually into a small bowl before you add them to the measuring cup. That way you don't accidentally get yolk into your already perfectly separated eggs. Save yolks for lemon curd.

To make meringues, mix egg whites and sugar and whisk in bowl of an electric mixer (if you have one) or in a large metal bowl. Place the bowl over simmering water (careful that the bottom isn't touching the water) and stir until sugar is dissolved for about 3 minutes. When you rub the mixture between your fingers it will be smooth and not grainy. Add cream of tartar. Attach bowl to the mixer, or using hand mixer, mix on highest speed until meringue is stiff and glossy. It should hold very stiff peaks when done. Using two tablespoons, scoop mounds of meringue onto sheet pan about 2" apart (they will expand as they bake). Use a spoon to pull peaks in the top of meringue mounds.

*continued on next page*

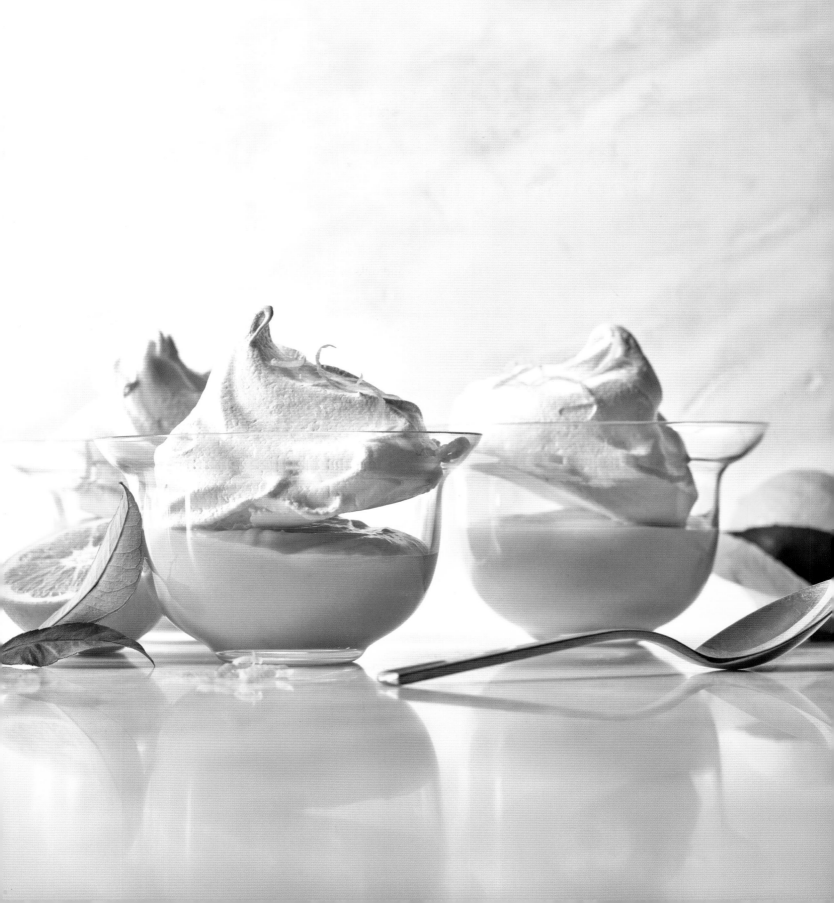

# chewy meringues & lemon curd *cont.*

Bake 25 minutes, rotating halfway through. Turn off oven and leave for 1½ hours in a warm oven to firm. Meringues can be made two days ahead of time and once completely cooled can be stored in an airtight container at room temperature.

While meringues are baking, prepare lemon curd. Place medium-sized metal bowl with yolks and sugar over a saucepan of simmering water (making sure water does not touch the bottom of the bowl). Whisk until sugar dissolves, about 3 minutes. Add juice and zest then whisk continuously until thickened, about 8–10 minutes. Curd will become light yellow in color, and when finished is the consistency of a soft pudding.

Remove from heat and whisk in ghee, one spoonful at a time, making sure each addition is melted before adding the next.

Using a rubber spatula, scoop into a glass container. A jar or glass dish works well. Lay plastic wrap directly onto the surface of the lemon curd.

To serve, place a large scoop of lemon curd into a small bowl and top with meringue.

# lemon granita

**MAKES 6 CUPS** | LF | V | GF

Here's an easy and tasty dessert. Leftovers can be frozen and broken up again when you are ready to eat.

### INGREDIENTS

Juice and zest from 5 lemons (about ½ cup)

½ cup sugar

5 cups hot water

### PREPARATION

Stir sugar and hot water together until sugar is dissolved. Bring to room temperature and add lemon juice and zest. Pour ingredients into a 9 × 13" baking dish. Place in the freezer for 3 hours. Every 30 minutes, use a fork to break up and scrape clumps of ice that begin to form.

# coconut custard flan

**MAKES 6 SERVINGS** | LF | V | GF
Adapted from *Natural Gourmet Institute*

Who knew a vegan, gluten-free flan made in under 30 minutes could be this delicious? It's a silken, creamy treat. If you don't have ramekins you can also make this in the cups of a muffin tin—a little harder to unmold but a workable solution.

## INGREDIENTS

### FOR FLAN:

3½ cups coconut milk
(two 13.5 oz cans)

2 tablespoon agar flakes
or 2 teaspoons agar powder

⅓ cup maple syrup

1 teaspoon vanilla extract

¼ teaspoon sea salt

1 tablespoon kuzu + 2 tablespoon water

### FOR CARAMEL SYRUP:

½ cup sugar

2 tablespoon water

## PREPARATION

Dissolve kuzu in water until there are no lumps. Add to milk mixture and simmer until slightly thickened, about 5 minutes.

Lightly oil ramekins with coconut oil. Pour coconut milk mixture into ramekins. Refrigerate to set.

When custard is set, run paring knife around the side of each ramekin to loosen. Invert custard onto plate, spooning any syrup left in ramekin over top of custard.

### CARAMEL SYRUP:

In a small, heavy-bottomed saucepan combine sugar and water until all the sugar is wet. Over medium heat, heat sugar without stirring until it becomes a light amber color about 15 minutes. Being very careful to not burn yourself, remove from heat and divide syrup evenly between ramekins. Do not touch the caramel with your fingers until completely cool. It is extraordinarily hot and hot sugar burns are no joke.

### FLAN:

In a medium-sized pot, combine coconut milk and agar. Soak agar for 5 minutes. Bring mixture to boil. Watch carefully as it will boil over quite quickly leaving you with a big mess on the stove. Reduce heat and simmer uncovered for about 5 minutes or more, until agar is completely dissolved. Add maple syrup, salt, and vanilla extract then stir until combined.

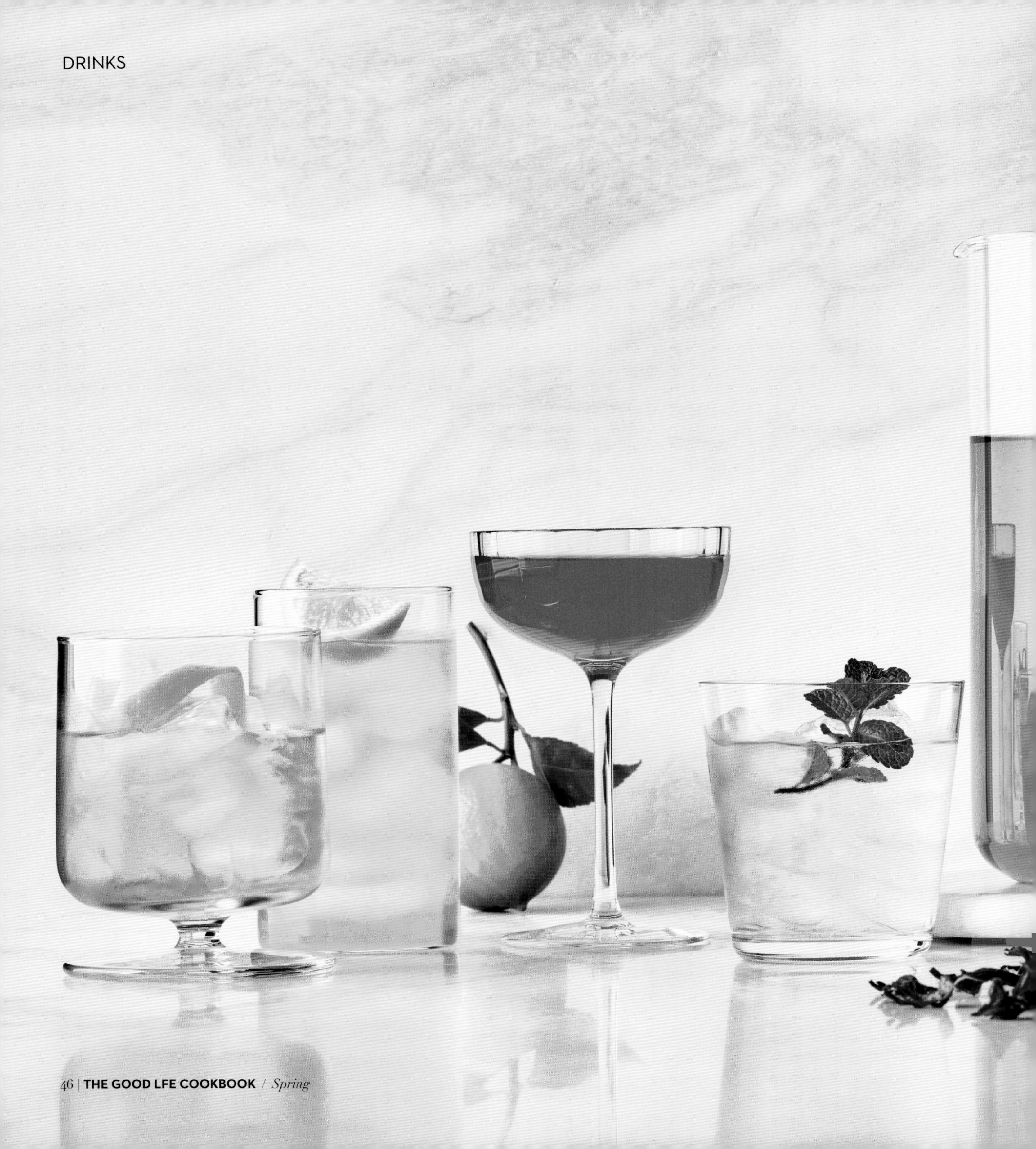

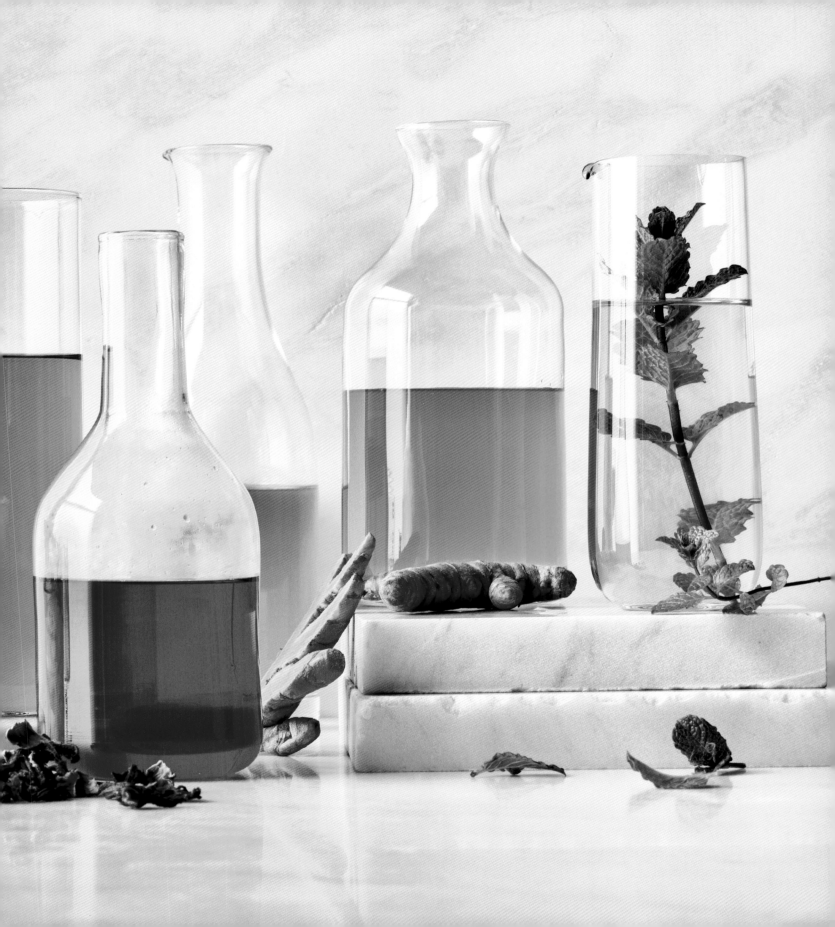

# lemongrass tea

**MAKES 1 QUART** | LF | V | GF

A bright lemon-flavored tea that makes a refreshing summer drink. Lemongrass is known for its anti-inflammatory, antimicrobial, and stomach-soothing properties. Fresh lemongrass can be found at Asian markets and most health food stores.

**INGREDIENTS**

5 stalks fresh lemongrass, roughly chopped or 5 tablespoons dried

1 quart water

**PREPARATION**

Bring water to a boil and simmer lemongrass for 5 minutes over medium-high heat. Remove from heat and let steep for an additional 5 minutes. Strain and chill. Can be refrigerated for up to 3 days.

# fresh mint tea

**MAKES 1 QUART** | LF | V | GF

Cooling and refreshing, this tea is quick enough to make by the cupful, but I like to make it by the quart so I have a go-to jar in the fridge.

**INGREDIENTS**

1 bunch fresh mint

1 quart boiling water

**PREPARATION**

Pour water over mint and let steep for 5 minutes. Strain.

# springtime nettle tea

**MAKES 1 QUART** | LF | V | GF

Fresh spring nettles are such a treat, but I often use dried nettles: they are more readily available and I don't have to wear gloves to handle them. Although nettle tea is available in bag form, which works in a pinch, I prefer to use loose nettles to make a stronger, overnight brew. It's high in vitamins A, C, and D. And it's full of minerals including magnesium, potassium, calcium, and zinc. I drink a cup of this tea daily throughout spring and summer.

**INGREDIENTS**

2 tablespoons dried nettles

1 quart boiling water

**PREPARATION**

Combine nettles and water in a quart jar and steep, covered, for 4 hours (or overnight). Strain. Can be refrigerated for up to 2 days.

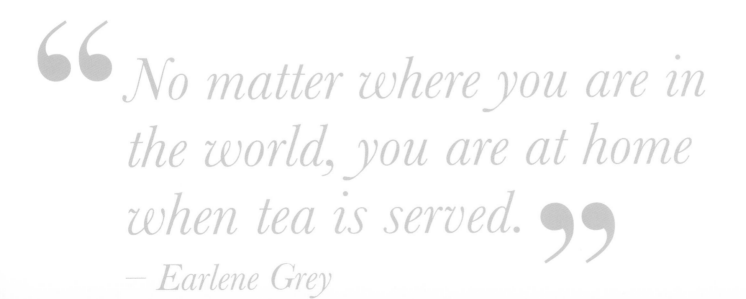

" *No matter where you are in the world, you are at home when tea is served.* "

— *Earlene Grey*

# simple margarita

**MAKES 1 COCKTAIL** | LF | V | GF

What you won't find in this recipe is Triple Sec—because it's loaded with sugar. The juice from a sweet, tangy orange and a bit of sugar essentially eliminates the need for the liqueur. This refreshing cocktail can be paired with Mexican flavors, or just about anything else.

### INGREDIENTS

Juice from 1 lime

Juice from 1 orange

Juice from ½ lemon

2 ounces tequila

1 tablespoon caster sugar

Lime slices, for serving

### PREPARATION

Shake all ingredients with ice in shaker. Serve on the rocks with a slice of lime.

# grapefruit mint caipiroska

**MAKES 1 COCKTAIL** | LF | V | GF

Based on a popular Brazilian cocktail, but made with vodka, the caipiroska has a lighter and more straightforward flavor profile. Don't skimp on the muddle, it's important to draw out the oils in the grapefruit and mint for a full hit of flavor.

### INGREDIENTS

¼ pink grapefruit cut into ¼" slices

1 sprig mint

2 teaspoons caster sugar

1 tablespoon water

2 ounces vodka

### PREPARATION

Muddle grapefruit, mint, and sugar in a rocks glass. Stir in water until sugar is dissolved. Add an ice cube and vodka and stir. Top off with ice and mint sprig.

# CHEERS! Enjoying cocktails while staying microbiome-balanced

*Alcohol can most certainly be part of a SIBO-friendly diet. It's important to note that some types of alcohol are better tolerated than others, so choose your mixers wisely or don't use them at all, and of course, enjoy in moderation.*

- Distilled spirits such as tequila and vodka are generally well-tolerated, and when enjoyed in moderation, do not upset the balance of the microbiome.

- Sugary mixers, highly carbonated beverages, and high-fructose corn syrup can wreak havoc on the system and should be avoided. That means no margaritas from pre-made mixers (see our SIBO-friendly recipe on the opposite page) .

- Watch out for mixers with unexpected additives. Most mass-market varieties of tonic water, for example, contain high-fructose corn syrup.

- Ideally, enjoy alcohol straight or combined with simple mixers, like seltzers and a squeeze of fresh lemon, lime, or other fresh fruit.

- When it comes to beer, the less hoppy, the better (for example, a lager or a pilsner is a better choice than an IPA).

- For individuals with SIBO who do not have IBS, both red and white wines are good choices. However, patients who also suffer from IBS often tolerate white wine better than red.

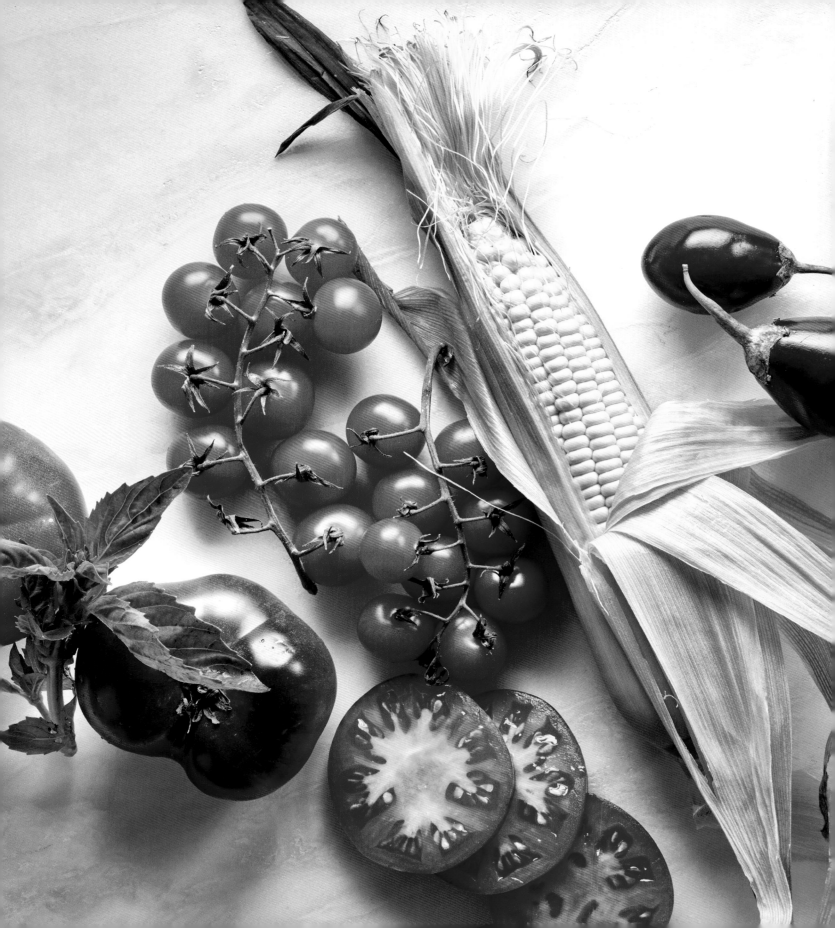

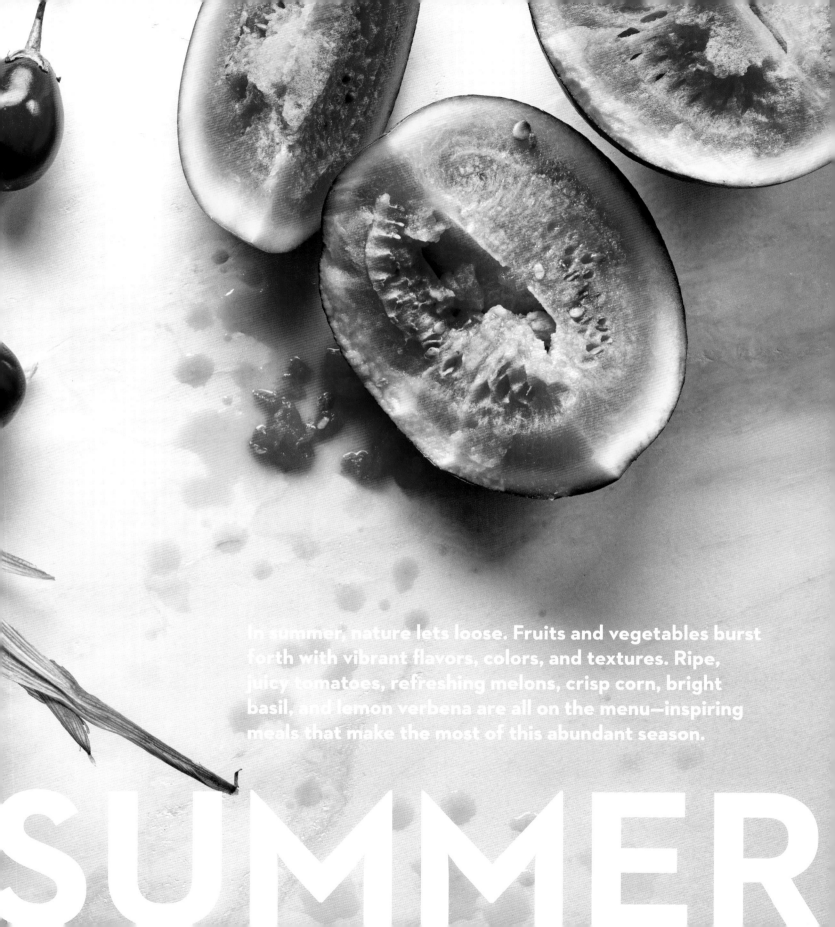

In summer, nature lets loose. Fruits and vegetables burst forth with vibrant flavors, colors, and textures. Ripe, juicy tomatoes, refreshing melons, crisp corn, bright basil, and lemon verbena are all on the menu—inspiring meals that make the most of this abundant season.

# SUMMER

With long days, warm nights, weekend getaways, and epic adventures, summer is the season where routines take a holiday and we let relaxation rule. Less stress is great for the microbiome, so say yes to relaxing backyard barbecues, picnics in the park, and dining al fresco. In the next pages, we'll show you just how easy it is to breeze through summer dining without a care, all while keeping your system in balance.

# zucchini muffins

**MAKES 9 MUFFINS** | LF | V
Adapted from *Smitten Kitchen*

These can also be made in a 8 × 4" loaf pan and baked for about an hour. It freezes well, so double the recipe if you want to save half for another time.

**INGREDIENTS**

2 eggs

½ cup olive oil

¾ cup turbinado sugar

1 teaspoon vanilla extract

Large pinch each: ginger, cardamom, cloves, nutmeg, cinnamon, coriander (no worries if you don't have all of these, just use what you have, equal to about a teaspoon)

½ teaspoon baking soda

¼ teaspoon baking powder

½ teaspoon salt

1 cup grated zucchini (about one small zucchini)

1 cup chopped pecans (optional)

1½ cups all-purpose flour

**PREPARATION**

Preheat oven to 350°F (180°C) and generously grease the muffin tins.

Whisk eggs, oil, sugar, and vanilla in a large bowl. Sprinkle spices, baking soda, baking powder, and salt over the top of wet ingredients and mix in well. Stir in zucchini and nuts (if using). Sprinkle flour over top and briefly stir until flour is incorporated.

Fill muffin tins ¾ of the way full and bake for 20–25 minutes (until toothpick stuck into center of muffin comes out clean), rotating halfway through.

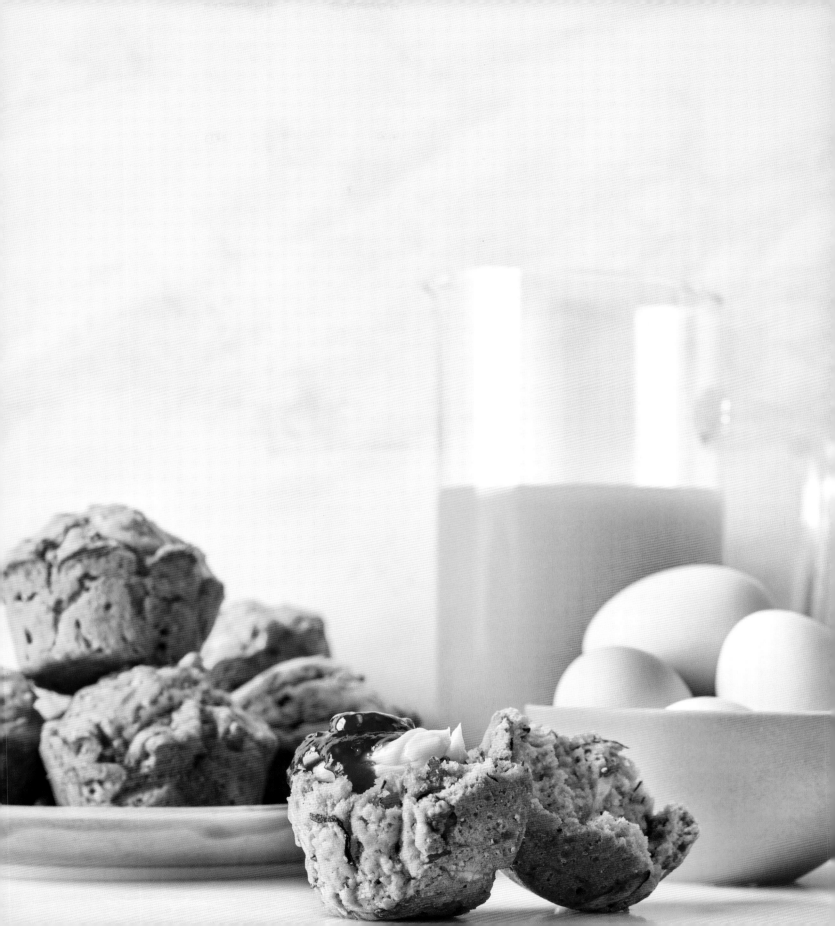

# roasted tomato & chard frittata

**MAKES 1 (12") FRITTATA** | LF | V | GF

There's a garden of goodness in this one-pan breakfast dish. Each serving delivers a healthy dose of vegetables and flavor, satisfying enough for any meal of the day.

## INGREDIENTS

1 pint cherry tomatoes, halved

1 bunch chard, stems removed and thinly sliced

Olive oil

2 cloves garlic, grated

1 cup Parmesan, grated

2 tablespoons thyme, chopped

### FOR EGGS:

12 eggs + 1 can (5.4 ounces) coconut cream + 1¼ teaspoon of salt blended in blender, or with hand blender, until frothy

## PREPARATION

Preheat oven to 400°F (200°C).

Toss cherry tomatoes with light coating of olive oil and roast, cut side up on a parchment-lined pan for 40 minutes until they are brown around edges and a little dry.

Sauté chard stems in a liberal amount of olive oil and a pinch of salt until tender, about five minutes. Add greens and cook until wilted and moisture is cooked out. Toss in garlic for last few minutes of cooking. Layer half of the Parmesan and tomatoes on top of greens and pour egg mixture over top. Top with remaining cheese, thyme, and tomatoes.

Cook over medium heat on stove until edges of frittata starts to set.

Bake at 400°F (200°C) for 15 minutes until middle of frittata is almost completely set. It will continue to firm up over next 10 minutes.

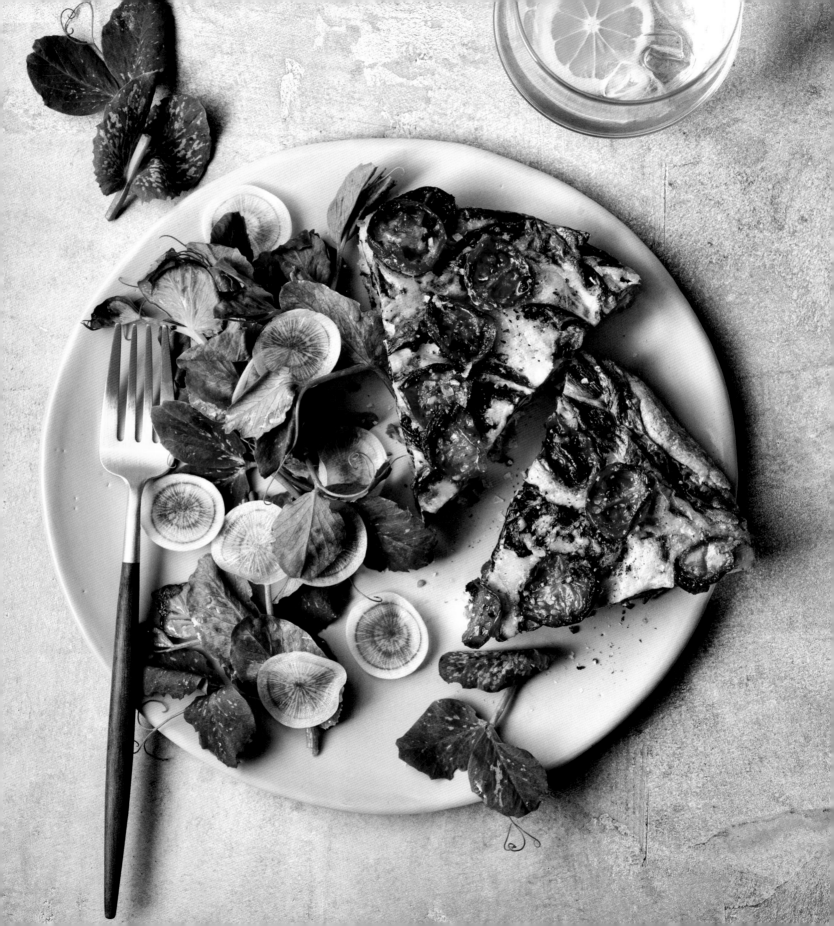

# deviled eggs *with* everything spice

**MAKES 2 DOZEN** | LF | V | GF

A brunch favorite, we keep them simple with a little touch of Everything Spice on top. The filling can be spooned or piped in. If you are making them ahead of time, keep the filling separate from the whites until the day you are serving them to keep the filling from getting runny.

## INGREDIENTS

12 eggs

1 tablespoon mayonnaise + more as needed

2 teaspoons mustard (Dijon will give you a spicy deviled egg, whole grain mustard will be more mild + more to taste, if needed)

½ teaspoon dry fine herbs (An herb blend of tarragon, chervil, chives, and parsley. Our favorite comes from Oaktown spice company. Herbs de Provence, dried tarragon and/or chives can also be used.)

Pinch paprika

Zest of 1 lemon

1 tablespoon Everything Spice

Cayenne, to taste

## PREPARATION

Start eggs in a large pot of boiling water and cook for 13 minutes, then plunge into ice bath until cooled.

Peel eggs and cut each egg in half, lengthwise. In a small bowl mash yolk with fork until very smooth. Add 1 tablespoon of mayonnaise and two teaspoons of mustard. Mix well. If yolks are still too dry add mayonnaise by the teaspoon. Season with herbs, paprika, and lemon zest, adding more to taste.

Fill whites with yolks either with piping bag or spoon. Sprinkle with Everything Spice and paprika before serving.

# prosciutto *with* melon

**MAKES 18 PIECES** | LF | GF

When cantaloupe is in season and ripe, this is one of the easiest and most delicious ways to enjoy it. The contrast of the salty ham and the sweet melon makes this a classic appetizer you'll serve over and over.

## INGREDIENTS

6 1" slices of cantaloupe, skin removed, cut into 3 pieces per slice

9 thin slices prosciutto (about ¼ pound), each slice torn in half

## PREPARATION

Wrap each piece of melon in a half-slice of prosciutto.

# corn cakes *with* cherry tomatoes

**MAKES 18 SMALL CAKES** | LF | V | GF

These are a lovely appetizer, cocktail party finger food, or a unique addition to a brunch menu. You can usually find corn flour in most health food stores or you can make your own by grinding cornmeal in your food processor until it is a fine powder. Using ghee to fry with adds flavor and the high smoke point keeps your kitchen from getting smoky.

## INGREDIENTS

¾ cups corn flour

Scant teaspoon baking powder

¼ teaspoon salt

2 pinches smoked paprika

2 eggs, separated

2 tablespoons butter or ghee, melted

½ cup almond, coconut, or lactose-free milk

1 cup corn kernels, fresh off the cob or frozen and defrosted

½ cup Gruyère cheese, grated

Ghee for pan

### GARNISH:

1 pint cherry tomatoes, quartered

Splash of red wine vinegar

Salt and ground black pepper, to taste

## PREPARATION

Mix dry ingredients together in a large bowl. Stir in egg yolks, butter, milk, corn, and cheese.

In a separate bowl or the bowl of a stand mixer, beat egg whites into stiff peaks and fold them into corn batter.

Heat a tablespoon of ghee in large skillet over medium heat. When pan is hot, drop scant tablespoons full into the hot oil. Push edges to create a round pancake. Cook for 3–4 minutes on each side until golden brown and a little crispy. Fry in batches adding more ghee to pan as needed.

Toss tomatoes, vinegar, salt and pepper together then garnish to top corn cakes. This dish is also delicious with smoked salmon.

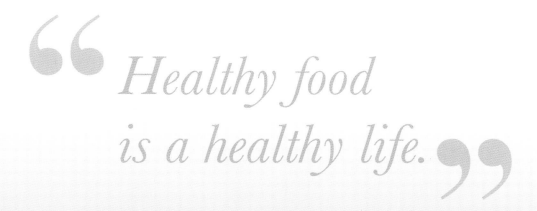

" *Healthy food is a healthy life.* "

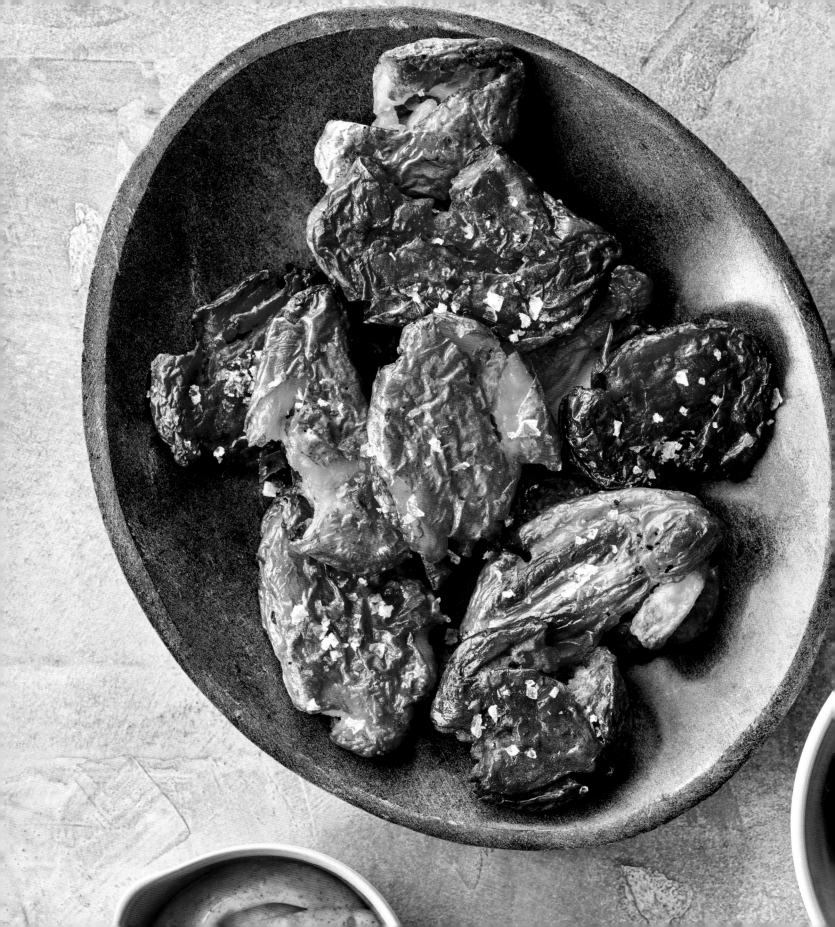

# crispy fingerling potatoes

**SERVES 6–8** | LF | V | GF

Boiling potatoes first gives the best of both worlds: creamy middles with crispy, crunchy outsides. Bake them within a few minutes of boiling and mash them to keep the insides from drying out. They are great on their own or served with Salsa Verde (p. 175) or Smoky Mayo (below) with Herb Salad (p. 22) piled on top.

**INGREDIENTS**

3 pounds fingerling potatoes, or large potatoes cut in half

4 tablespoons olive oil

Salt

**PREPARATION**

Preheat oven to 450°F (230°C). Put potatoes in a large pot of salted cold water, bring to a boil and cook until potatoes are tender, about 20–30 minutes. Drain and toss hot potatoes in two tablespoons of olive oil and two generous pinches of salt.

Spread potatoes out on a large parchment-lined sheet pan with plenty of space between each potato. With a potato masher, smash potato until split open and slightly flattened. Drizzle smashed potatoes with remaining olive oil and a sprinkle of salt then roast for 20–30 minutes until tops and edges of potatoes are crispy, flipping over halfway through.

# smoky mayo

**MAKES ½ CUP** | LF | V | GF

Something quick and easy to whip up as a spread for burgers or a dip for potatoes.

**INGREDIENTS**

½ cup mayonnaise

1½ teaspoons mild smoked paprika

½ teaspoon red vinegar

Pinch of salt

**PREPARATION**

Mix all ingredients together and season to taste. If you like it spicier, add a pinch of cayenne or dash of hot sauce to taste.

# baked tortilla chips

**MAKES 4–6 DOZEN CHIPS** | LF | V | GF

I have always been skeptical of baked chips but these are *just as good* as fried chips and use much less oil. They're healthier and your kitchen stays tidy.

### INGREDIENTS

1 package good quality
corn tortillas

¼ cup neutral oil like avocado,
grapeseed, or sunflower

Salt, to taste

### PREPARATION

Preheat oven to 425°F (220°C). Place your unwrapped tortillas on a cutting board. Brush one tortilla with oil on both sides. Stack another tortilla on top. Brush the top of the tortilla you placed on top. Continue stacking and brushing all tortillas.

Cut the stack of tortillas into 8 triangular pieces, like a stack of tiny pizzas. Lay oiled tortillas on a parchment-lined sheet pan making sure they don't overlap. You may need to use 2 sheet pans. Sprinkle with a few pinches of salt.

Bake chips for 12–18 minutes until completely crispy all the way through. If your oven heats up evenly, you may not have to flip them halfway through. Just check to make sure the bottoms aren't browning too quickly. They should be very slightly golden but not brown.

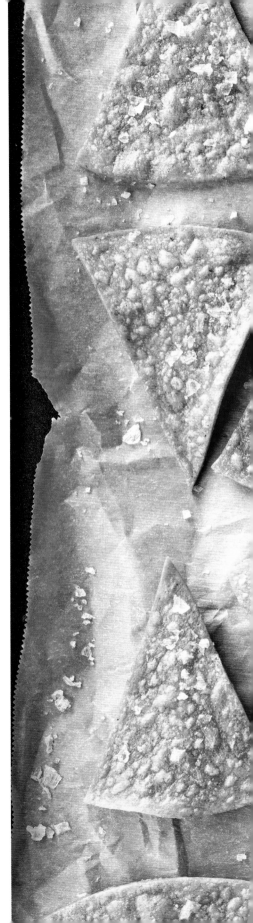

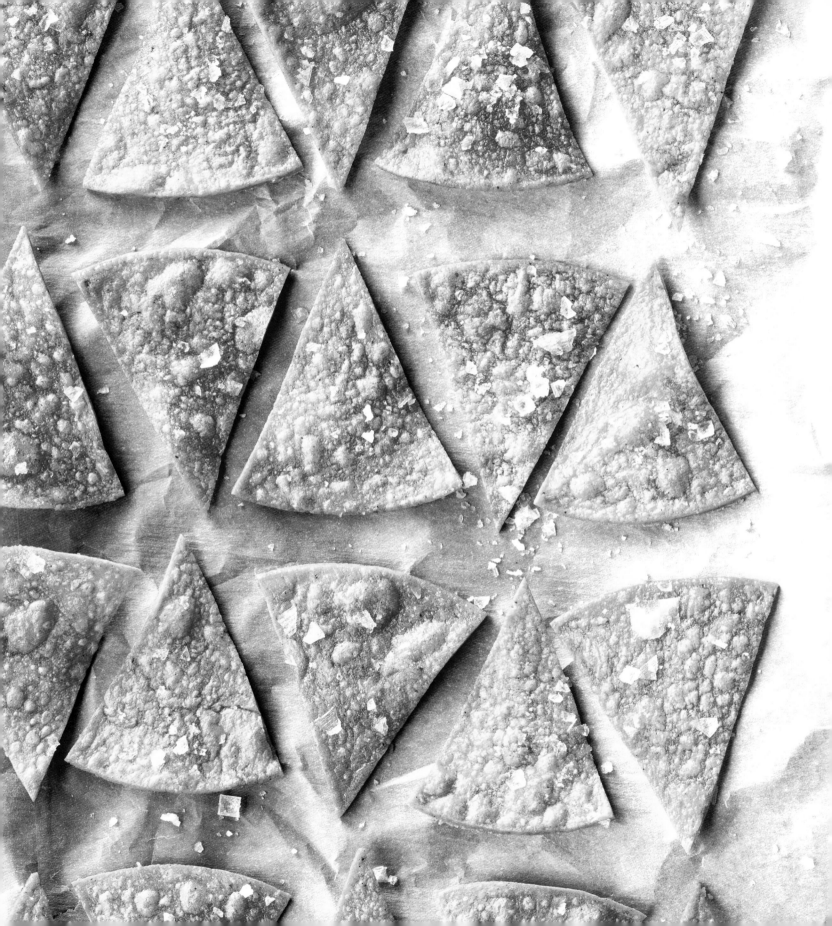

# mango salsa

**MAKES 1 ½ CUPS** | LF | V | GF

This is summer in a bowl. It balances the richness of meat dishes, like pulled pork, and pairs wonderfully with a simple grilled or pan fried fish. It's also completely acceptable to eat it out of the bowl with crispy tortilla chips or a spoon.

**INGREDIENTS**

1 mango, cut into small cubes

½ bell pepper, diced

3 scallions, thinly sliced

Large handful cilantro leaves, minced

Juice and zest of 1 lime

Large pinch cayenne

Sea salt and ground black pepper, to taste

**PREPARATION**

Combine all ingredients in a large bowl. Season with lime, cayenne, salt and pepper to taste.

# restaurant style tomato salsa

**MAKES 3 CUPS** | LF | V | GF

I have made salsa with fresh tomatoes and tomatoes I roasted myself, but I have found that using a jar of my Simple Summertime Tomato Sauce (p. 79) or a can of diced tomatoes creates a salsa like what's served at the neighborhood Mexican restaurant.

**INGREDIENTS**

1 red onion

3 cloves garlic

Large handful cilantro leaves

1 pint of Simple Summertime Tomato Sauce (p. 79) or 1 can (14 ounces) of organic diced tomatoes

Salt and ground black pepper, to taste

1 chipotle chili from can of adobo, or 1 jalapeño, seeded and roasted on sheet pan with onions + pinch of smoked paprika

Juice of 1 lime

**PREPARATION**

Preheat oven to 500°F (260°C). Cut onion into large chunks and scatter onto parchment-lined sheet pan with peeled garlic cloves and a generous drizzle of olive oil. Roast for 15 minutes until onions and garlic are soft and slightly charred. Place in food processor with remaining ingredients.

Pulse until cilantro and onions are finely chopped. Season to taste with salt, pepper, chile pepper, and lime.

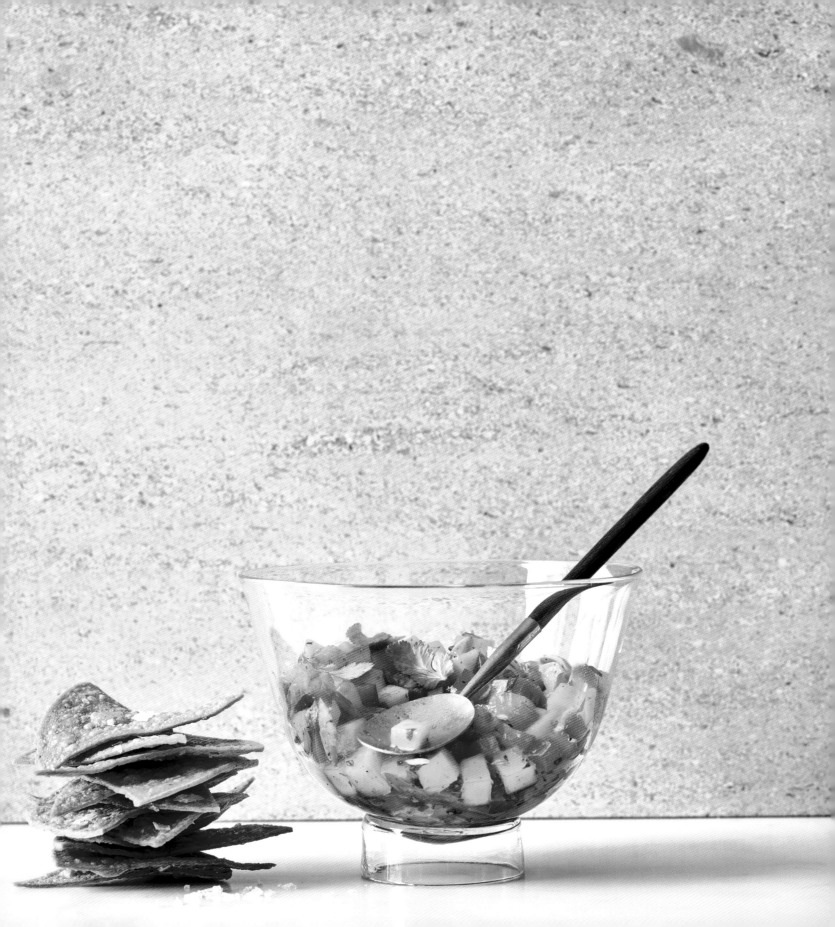

# green goddess dressing

**MAKES 2/3 CUP** | LF | V | GF

Green goddess dressing slathered on little gem lettuce and sprinkled with toasted hazelnuts is a salad favorite for us. This dressing is also fantastic as a spread on grilled vegetable sandwiches, chicken sandwiches made with leftover roasted chicken, or as a dip for crudité.

### INGREDIENTS

2 avocados, sliced and skins removed

Handful each of parsley, basil, tarragon, chives, and mint

Juice and zest of 1 lemon

White wine vinegar

Olive oil

Salt and ground black pepper, to taste

### PREPARATION

Place avocados, herbs, lemon juice and zest into a small food processor or blender. Blend until smooth, adding olive oil as needed to get a creamy dressing. Season to taste with vinegar, salt and pepper.

# carrot ginger dressing

**1 1/2 CUPS** | LF | V | GF

Try this nutrient-dense dressing for salads. As a post-workout snack, top half an avocado with a tablespoon of this tasty dressing.

### INGREDIENTS

3 carrots, roughly chopped

1 stalk celery, roughly chopped

1/4 shallot

1 1/2" piece of ginger, peeled

1/8 cup rice vinegar

1 teaspoon dry mustard

Pinch white pepper

Salt to taste

1/2 cup neutral oil, like avocado, grapeseed, or sunflower

1/2 teaspoon tahini

Water as needed

### PREPARATION

Purée carrots, celery, shallot, and ginger in food processor with vinegar and spices. With food processor running at low speed, add oil and tahini. If too thick, add water to the purée by the tablespoon until dressing is thinned to desired consistency.

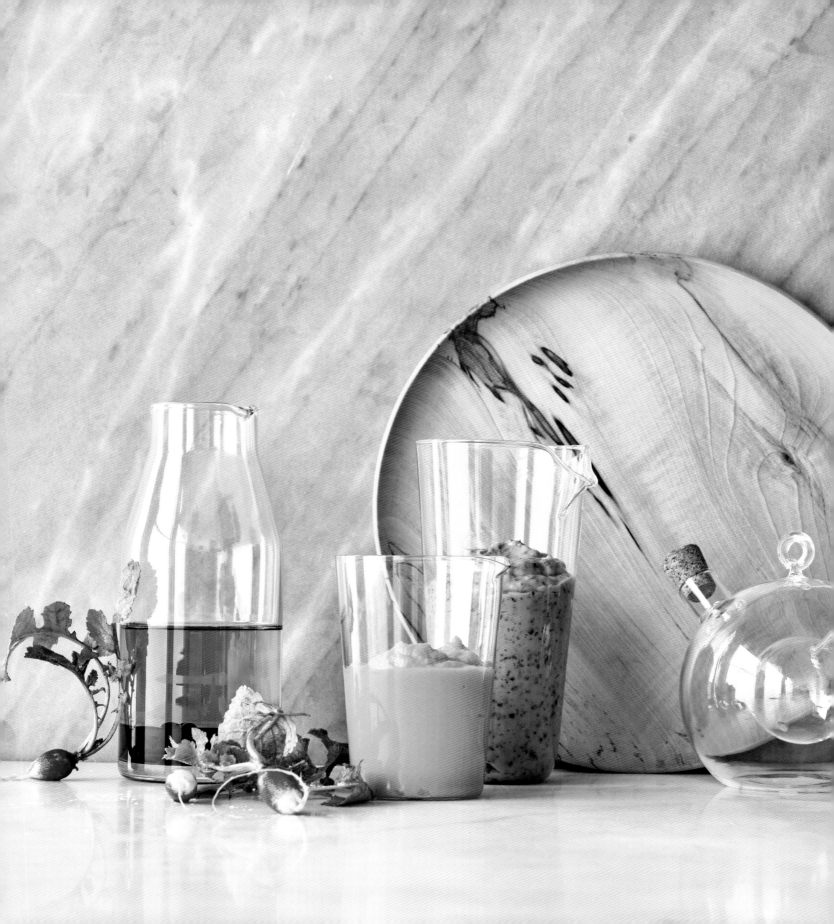

# balsamic vinaigrette

**MAKES ABOUT ¾ CUP** | LF | V | GF

Consider this dressing an essential at mealtime. Making this zingy dressing in a pinch is a skill you'll want to have, and with the abundance of salad greens in summer, you'll have plenty of practice.

### INGREDIENTS

⅓ cup garlic-infused olive oil, or plain olive oil

⅓ cup balsamic vinegar

1 teaspoon honey

1 teaspoon Dijon mustard

½ teaspoon sea salt

¼ teaspoon ground black pepper

### PREPARATION

Put all ingredients in a jar and shake until combined.

# caesar dressing

**MAKES 1 CUP** | LF | GF

This dressing is a little lighter and fresher than your typical creamy Caesar dressings. Start with one garlic clove and then add more if you want a bit of a kick. The flavors come together after a day in the refrigerator, so make this a day ahead. This dressing and crispy romaine with leftover roasted chicken is a lunchtime favorite.

### INGREDIENTS

1 small garlic clove, grated with a microplane

3 anchovy fillets

1 teaspoon Dijon mustard

Zest of 1 lemon

Juice of 1 lemon

½ teaspoon Lord Sandy's Worcestershire Sauce or coconut aminos

2 tablespoons parsley, minced

¼ cup Parmesan cheese, finely grated

3 tablespoons olive oil

3 tablespoons grapeseed or avocado oil

Salt and ground black pepper, to taste

### PREPARATION

With the back of a fork, mash garlic and anchovy fillets into a paste with a pinch of salt. Add Dijon and lemon zest and continue to mash into a paste. Whisk in lemon juice, Worcestershire sauce or coconut aminos, parsley, cheese, and several grinds of fresh pepper.

Slowly whisk in oils. Season to taste.

# greek salad

**MAKES 8 CUPS** | LF | V | GF

Herbs, ripe summer tomatoes, and a bright fresh marinade make this one of my go-to summer salads. Letting it sit before serving gives the vegetables time to marinate.

## INGREDIENTS

1 shallot or ½ red onion, thinly sliced in ¼ moons and soaked in 2 tablespoons red wine vinegar (optional)

2 English cucumbers, cut into ½" quarter moons

2 red bell peppers

1 pint cherry tomatoes or four medium-sized tomatoes

¼ cup parsley, minced

¼ cup mint, minced

2 tablespoons oregano, minced

½ cup Kalamata olives, pitted and torn in half

2 teaspoons sumac

Juice and zest of 1 lemon

3 tablespoons olive oil

Salt and ground black pepper, to taste

## PREPARATION

When shallot (or onion) is bright pink after soaking in red wine vinegar for about 15 minutes, toss all ingredients in a large bowl. Season to taste with salt and pepper. Let sit for 15–30 minutes at room temperature before serving.

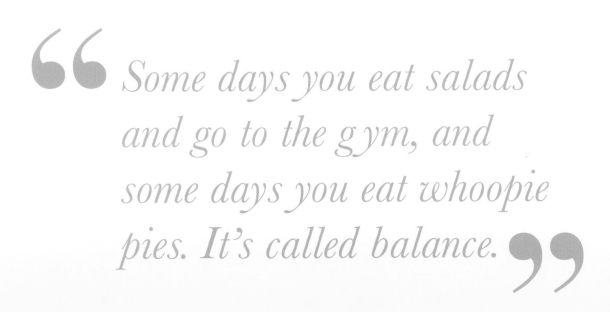

*" Some days you eat salads and go to the gym, and some days you eat whoopie pies. It's called balance. "*

# heirloom tomato & arugula salad

**SERVES 6-8** | LF | V | GF

This is an ode to the last of the season's tomatoes.

### INGREDIENTS

1 bag (8 ounces) baby arugula

3–4 medium/large heirloom tomatoes, sliced (about 1 pound)

½ cup pine nuts, toasted

Balsamic Vinaigrette (p. 70)

Herbed Bread Crumbs (optional, p. 175)

### PREPARATION

On a large serving platter, layer the baby arugula, followed by the tomatoes, and then pine nuts.

Whisk together the vinaigrette ingredients in a small bowl and pour over tomatoes and arugula. Top with a sprinkling of Herbed Bread Crumbs for added crunch.

# tomato basil panzanella

**SERVES 6-8** | LF | V

This popular Tuscan salad made of tomatoes and crunchy bread is a summer delight. The fresh flavors and textures are simply wonderful. Serve as a side or a light meal on its own. Allow a little time at the end to let the liquids absorb into the bread.

### INGREDIENTS

½ round sourdough loaf or 1 sourdough baguette, cut or ripped into 1" cubes

1 shallot, thinly sliced

Balsamic Vinaigrette (p. 70)

2 pints cherry tomatoes, halved or 5 large heirloom tomatoes cut into 2" pieces

1 bunch basil, chopped

Salt and ground black pepper, to taste

### PREPARATION

Preheat oven to 350°F (180°C). Cut or tear bread into 1" cubes, toss with olive oil and spread into a single layer on parchment-lined sheet pan. Bake for 15 minutes and turn over and bake for another 15 minutes (or until crispy).

While croutons are toasting, marinate shallots in Balsamic Vinaigrette for 15 minutes. Toss tomatoes with marinated shallots, basil, a few spoonfuls of vinaigrette, and salt and pepper to taste. Toss in croutons and add dressing. Let sit for 10 minutes before serving.

# watermelon & basil salad

**SERVES 6-8** | LF | V | GF

Bright and refreshing, this salad can be served as a starter or dessert.

---

### INGREDIENTS

2 small seedless watermelons or 1 medium watermelon (about 3½–4 pounds)

8 sprigs each mint and basil, leaves picked and chiffonaded

Juice and zest of 2 limes

1 tablespoon olive oil

### PREPARATION

Cut off ends of watermelon and use knife to remove rind. Cut into 1" cubes. Toss watermelon with herbs, lime juice and zest, and olive oil.

*You say tomato, we say anti-inflammatory, hydrating, cancer-fighting, and a delicious SIBO-friendly powerhouse...*

## SLICED, DICED, OR SAUTÉED, THEIR NUTRITION SHINES THROUGH

Not only do tomatoes add a note of freshness to any dish, they deliver a boost of lycopene any way they're served. Unlike some vegetables whose potency can diminish when cooked, sautéeing tomatoes in olive oil or other heart-friendly oils breaks down the tomatoes' cellular walls, which actually increases lycopene's bioavailability. Lycopene and olive oil are both fat-soluble, so served in combination they help improve absorption of this powerful carotenoid. Lycopene, an antioxidant, also has anti-inflammatory, cancer-preventing, and vision-supporting properties. That's wonderful news to us. As much as we appreciate eating a ripe tomato plucked freshly off the vine, we can't resist adding a generous drizzle of olive oil, and maybe even a light sprinkle of shiso salt, while you're at it. Healthy never tasted so good.

# thai zucchini salad

**SERVES 6** | LF | V | GF

This is a mix between pad Thai and a salad. Use all zucchini noodles or half-zucchini and half-rice noodles, whichever you prefer. Add grilled shrimp or chicken on top to make it a complete meal.

### INGREDIENTS

3 zucchini, made into noodles with spiralizer, or 1 zucchini and 1 smallbundle rice noodles cooked as directed on package

2 carrots, julienned or made into noodles

1 red bell pepper, julienned

1 pint cherry tomatoes, cut into quarters, reserve some for garnish

Handful of green beans, steamed and cut into 1" pieces

Handful of basil, chiffonaded

Handful of cilantro, picked off stems

1 cup peanuts, toasted and chopped

Lime juice

Salt

### PREPARATION

Toss all vegetables and herbs together with enough Peanut Sauce (below) to lightly coat everything. Season to taste with lime and salt. Top with peanuts and tomatoes.

# peanut sauce

**MAKES 1 ½ cups** | LF | V | GF

With a few simple ingredients, this no-cook sauce packs a punch of peanut flavor. And you won't have to use the stovetop, heating up the kitchen, to make it. Tweak the flavors to your liking and serve as a dip or with cooked meats, vegetables, or vegetable noodles.

### INGREDIENTS

1 can (5.4 ounces) coconut cream or same amount of coconut milk

½ cup peanut butter

2 tablespoons coconut aminos

1 tablespoon rice vinegar

Juice of 1 lime + more to taste

½ teaspoon ginger, dried or fresh grated

½ teaspoon white pepper

5 dried kaffir lime leaves

1 teaspoon lemongrass, dried or fresh

Chili flakes or Sriracha chili sauce, to taste

Maple syrup, agave, honey, or brown sugar, to taste

Salt, to taste

### PREPARATION

Place all ingredients in food processor and blend until smooth. Season with sweetener, lime juice, salt, and chili, to taste.

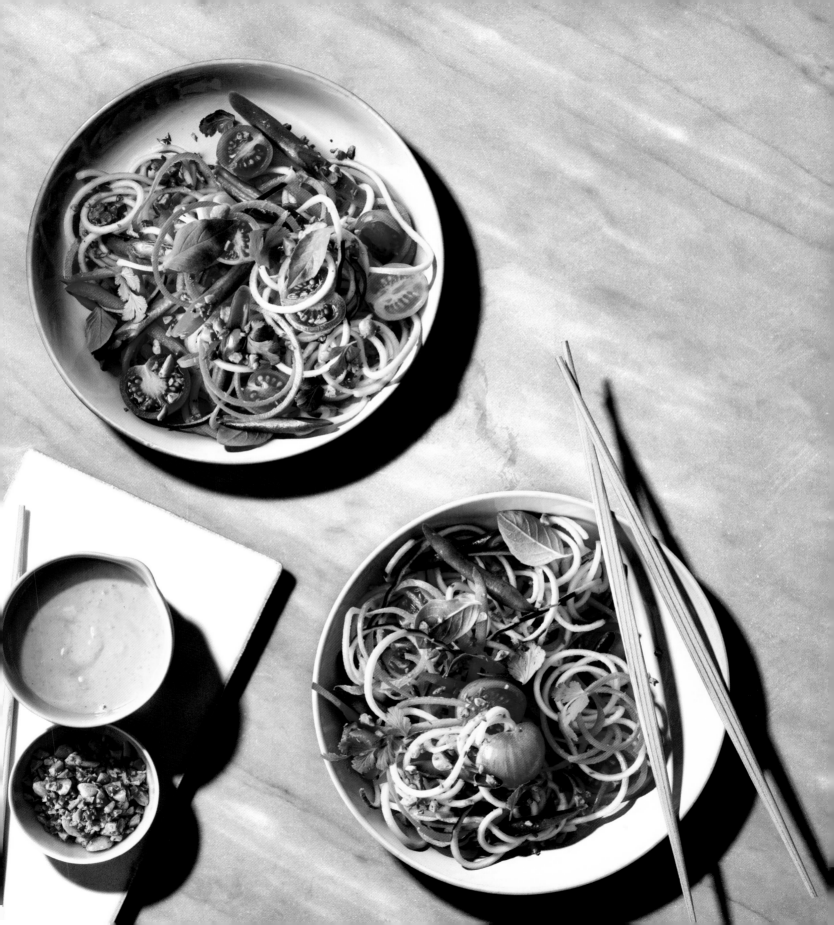

# grilled vegetable salad

**SERVES 6-8** | LF | V | GF

Whenever we grill outside, we always throw extra vegetables onto the grill, toss with a Dijon or balsamic dressing and serve with whatever else we are grilling. Feel free to use whatever vegetables you have on hand. We sometimes toss scallions, red onions and/or portobello mushrooms into the mix.

## INGREDIENTS

1 large eggplant, cut into ¼" slices

2 zucchini, cut lengthwise into ½" slices

2 summer squash, cut lengthwise into ½" slices

1 red bell pepper, cut into 1" slices

1 yellow bell pepper, cut into 1" slices

2 bulbs fennel, cut into ½" slices

### GARNISH WITH:

1 pint cherry tomatoes, quartered (do not grill)

2 tablespoons basil, tarragon or parsley, chopped

## PREPARATION

Toss cut vegetables in whatever dressing you are using and lay onto grill. Fennel, eggplant, and bell pepper will take about 4–6 minutes on each side. Zucchini and summer squash will take about 3 minutes on each side. I usually keep an eye on them and take them off the grill when they are cooked through but not yet mushy. Transfer to a platter with tongs as they finish.

When all the vegetables are cooked and laid out on your platter, toss with dressing and herbs, season with salt and pepper, and top with tomatoes.

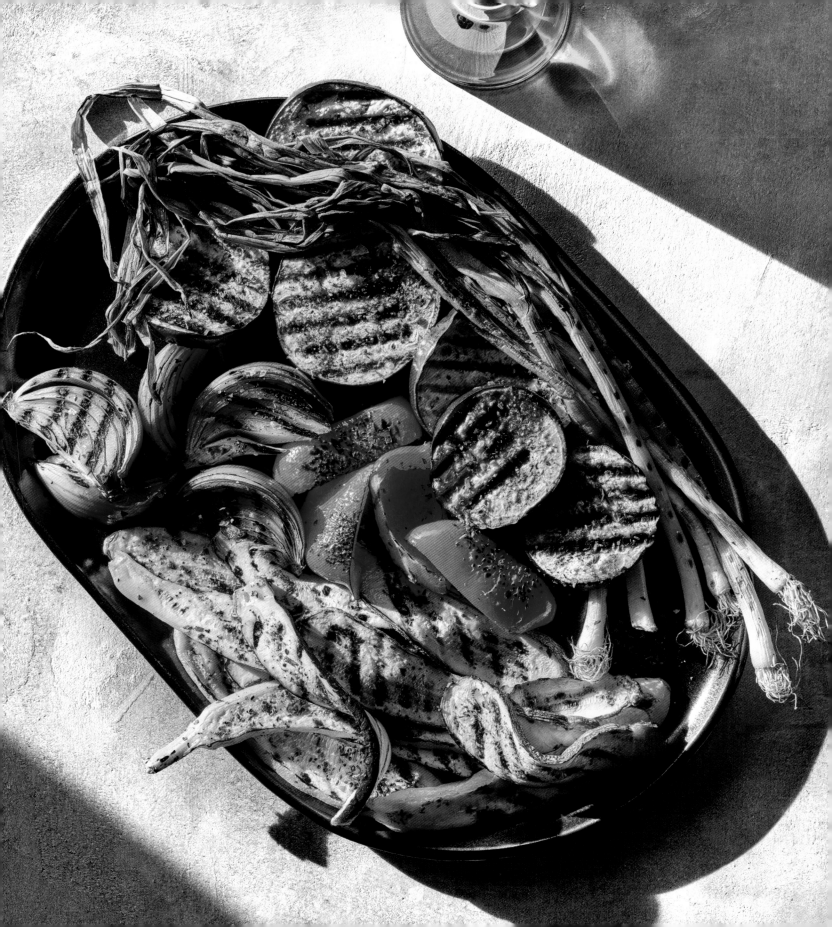

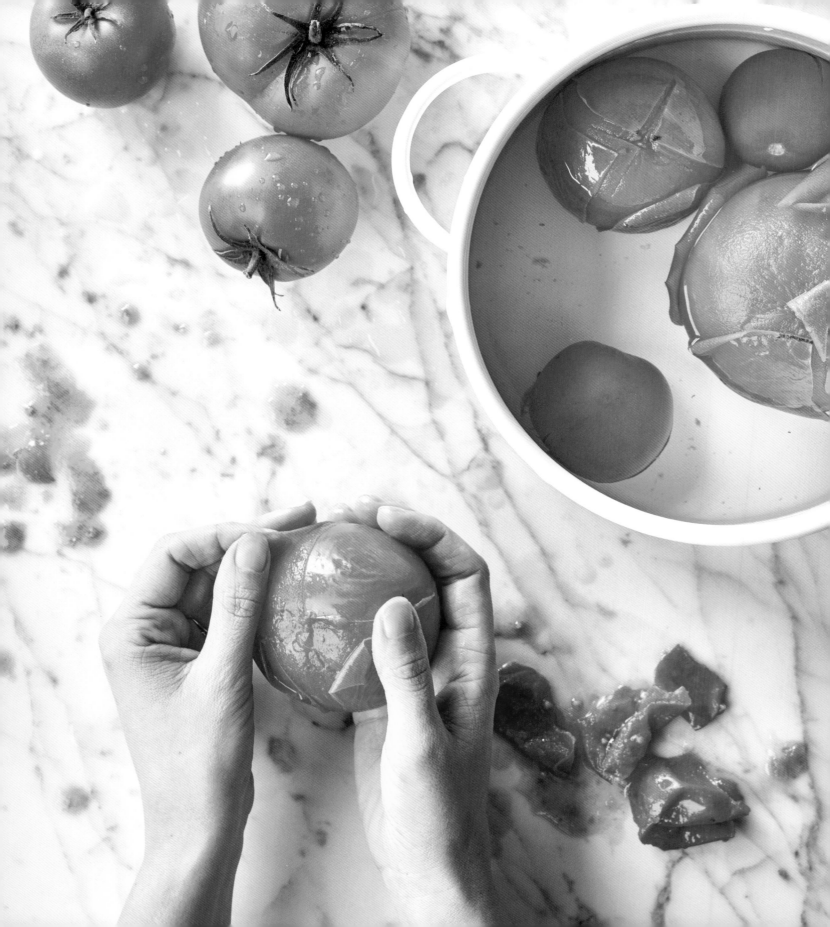

# simple summertime tomato sauce

**MAKES 2 QUARTS** | LF | V | GF

There are so many excellent canned tomatoes available these days but in New York City during the dog days of summer, I take advantage of the abundance of ripe tomatoes and make several quarts of tomato sauce to keep in the freezer. Defrosting a jar of sauce makes for a sunny treat in the middle of the gray slushy winter when I fantasize about living in Los Angeles (this happens every year in the middle of February and then subsides as everything thaws in May). The yellow heirloom tomatoes mixed with red tomatoes make a lovely orange sauce but any variety of ripe tomato will do. I find that it is worth it to spend the time and money and double or triple the batch, as it is satisfying to have quarts to stash away and only have to clean up the tomato mess once.

### INGREDIENTS

10 ripe heirloom and beefsteak tomatoes or 20 smaller tomatoes like Romas or San Marzanos (about 5 pounds)

¾ cup dry white wine (optional)

Salt, to taste

### PREPARATION

Fill a large stockpot of water ⅔ full and bring to a light boil. While water is heating, slice a shallow X on the bottom of each tomato with a sharp paring knife. Using tongs, gently lower 5–10 tomatoes into the hot water. Make sure they have enough room to float around a little bit so the skin will be loosened evenly all the way around. Blanch for about 3 minutes. You will be able to see the skin peeling back. Use tongs to lift them out of the water into a bowl (be careful, they are slippery).

Let cool for 5–10 minutes or until cool to the touch; the skin should slide right off. After peeling use a small, sharp paring knife to remove the core (slide knife in about ½" at a 45° angle and turn knife in a circle around top of core). I like to do this over the pot I will be cooking in to catch any of the juice. Use a potato masher to break tomatoes up into a rough, chunky sauce.

Place mashed tomatoes on stove over medium heat and bring to a low simmer. Add wine, if using, and let it cook out until it no longer smells like alcohol. Use a potato masher to break up any remaining large chunks. Simmer for 45 minutes. At this point you should have a nice consistency. Feel free to cook longer if you like a thicker sauce. Ladle into clean jars. The sauce will keep in the freezer for several months or in the refrigerator for about a week. When reheating, add olive oil, a grated garlic clove, and salt and herbs, to taste.

# orzo *with* spinach & roasted tomatoes

**MAKES 5 CUPS** | LF | V | GF

Bright and flavorful, this is the perfect partner to a roasted fish, or on its own with a spinach salad for a light lunch.

## INGREDIENTS

1 pint cherry tomatoes, halved

Sea salt

Olive oil

2 cups orzo pasta

4 tablespoons garlic-infused olive oil, divided

3 cloves thinly sliced garlic

12 ounces baby spinach

Zest of 1 lemon

¼ cup lemon juice

¾ cup finely grated Parmesan cheese

¼ cup tightly packed parsley leaves, minced

½ cup pine nuts, toasted

Salt and ground black pepper, to taste

## PREPARATION

Set an oven rack to the highest position and preheat to 400°F (200°C). Toss cherry tomatoes with a pinch of sea salt and 2 teaspoons olive oil. Transfer to a parchment-lined sheet pan and roast on the top rack for 40 minutes. Switch the oven to broil and broil for 1 minute to slightly char the tomatoes.

While the tomatoes are cooking, fill a medium-sized pot with water, add a large pinch of salt, and bring water to a boil. Add orzo and cook, stirring occasionally, for 7–9 minutes or according to package instructions. Strain and set aside.

Heat a sauté pan over medium-high heat. Add 1 tablespoon garlic-infused olive oil. Sauté spinach along with a pinch of salt and cook until wilted. Remove spinach from pan and sauté garlic in 1 tablespoon of oil until fragrant.

In a large bowl, combine orzo, sautéed spinach, roasted tomatoes, garlic, lemon zest and juice, Parmesan cheese, parsley, pine nuts, and two large pinches of salt and pepper. Adjust salt and lemon, to taste.

# balsamic chicken

**SERVES 6–8** | LF | V | GF

This chicken recipe is great to make for dinner and then use the leftovers the next day for lunch in a salad or sandwich. I prefer chicken thighs as they are a little more flavorful but you can also use breasts. When using marinades in sauces, make sure you bring to a boil and simmer vigorously for at least 5 minutes to make sure any juices from the meat are thoroughly cooked.

## INGREDIENTS

8 whole boneless skinless breasts, or 10 boneless skinless thighs

½ cup olive oil

⅔ cup balsamic vinegar

1 tablespoon each of rosemary, thyme, sage, oregano, chopped

Salt and ground black pepper, to taste

## PREPARATION

Place chicken in a baking dish and season with herbs and salt and pepper. Add the olive oil and balsamic vinegar and mix to coat. Marinate for 30 minutes–3 hours.

Cook in large skillet over medium-high heat until browned on both sides. Add marinade to pan, bring to boil, then reduce heat and simmer for 5 minutes more until chicken is cooked through and marinade is reduced by half.

## THE IMPORTANCE OF HEALTHY PORTIONS

What you eat is important, but so is the amount you eat. Too much of even the healthiest foods can put a strain on the digestive system, leading to discomfort for just about anyone. But for someone with SIBO or other gastrointestinal conditions, an overloaded system can cause issues that take several hours, if not days, to put back in balance. Portion control is tricky because there's no one-size-fits-all answer. The right portion for you depends on several factors, including age, gender, health needs, metabolism, activity level, and myriad other factors. Your best option is to work with a physician, dietitian, or nutritionist to determine the portions right for your needs. If that's not an option, search online for guidance from a well-respected medical institution.

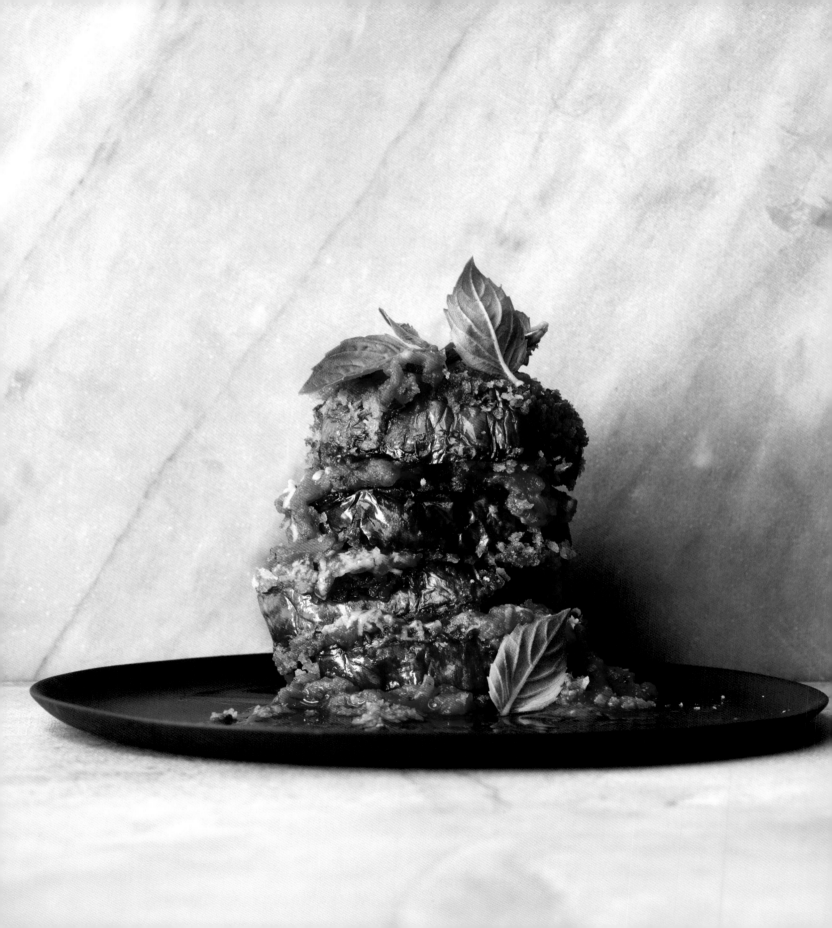

# eggplant parmesan

**SERVES 4–8** | LF | V | GF

Satisfying and cozy, top this dish with bread crumbs or almond flour to make a crisp coating on the outside of your eggplant before baking.

## INGREDIENTS

### SAUCE:

4 cups Simple Summertime Tomato Sauce (p. 79) or 2 large cans of organic diced tomatoes

6 garlic cloves, grated

2 teaspoon sugar

3 tablespoons oregano, chopped

1 teaspoon salt

Ground black pepper, to taste

### EGGPLANT:

2 large purple or confetti eggplant, sliced lengthwise into ¼" slices and salted for 30 minutes

2 cups bread crumbs or almond flour, seasoned with salt, pepper, and 2 tablespoons Italian herbs

1 cup rice or all-purpose flour, seasoned with salt and pepper

3 eggs, beaten and seasoned with salt and pepper

½ cup grapeseed, avocado, or other neutral oil with high smoke point

### TO FINISH:

2 cups grated Parmesan

½ cup basil, chiffonaded

## PREPARATION

To make the sauce combine all ingredients in a medium saucepan and bake at 500°F (260°C) for 30 minutes, until reduced by half. If it seems too thick to ladle onto the eggplant, add a few tablespoons of water. Season to taste. Reduce oven to 350°F (180°C).

While sauce is cooking fill three plates: one with flour, one with bread crumbs, and one with eggs. Press eggplant with paper towels to remove any excess water. Line a baking sheet with paper towels for cooked eggplant. Dip each slice into egg, then flour, back to egg and then into bread crumbs. I like to do this while I heat ¼ cup oil in a large skillet and drop each piece into the skillet as I make them. This saves you from dirtying another dish. Or, you can lay the coated eggplant onto a sheet pan and cook once they are all battered.

Fry each slice of eggplant until cooked through and golden brown on both sides, then lay on sheet pan lined with paper towel. When all slices are fried, ladle a light layer of cooked tomato sauce on the bottom of baking dish. Add layer of eggplant on top, then another ladle of sauce and a handful of cheese. Repeat until all the eggplant is in baking dish then top with cheese.

Bake at 350°F (180°C) for 20 minutes until cheese is bubbly and brown. Top with fresh basil.

If you like, add a layer of wilted spinach between each layer of eggplant.

# turkey burger *with* special sauce

**MAKES 6–8 BURGERS** | LF | GF

These burgers have some hidden vegetables to balance your meat intake and increase your vegetable servings. Grated vegetables also help to keep your burgers from drying out. The bread crumbs help to keep them in one piece, as turkey burgers tend to be more crumbly than beef burgers. If you can't find ground dark meat turkey you can add a tablespoon of olive oil to add the extra fat that the white meat lacks.

### INGREDIENTS

1 zucchini, finely grated

1 carrot, finely grated

¼ red onion, finely grated

1 egg

1 teaspoon salt

½ teaspoon pepper

1 teaspoon paprika

3 tablespoon bread crumbs or almond flour, more if needed

1 pound ground dark meat turkey

### SPECIAL SAUCE:

½ cup mayonnaise

¼ cup yellow mustard

2 tablespoons ketchup (free from corn syrup)

2 tablespoons sweet relish

¼ white onion, minced

1 teaspoon onion powder

2½ teaspoons paprika

### PREPARATION

Wrap zucchini and carrot in a clean kitchen towel and squeeze to remove excess moisture. In a medium-sized bowl, mix vegetables, eggs, salt, pepper, paprika, and bread crumbs (if using)until well combined. Gently mix in meat until combined.

Divide mixture into 6 balls. In a large skillet over medium-high heat, place two of the meatballs into the pan and smash with the back of a spatula until flattened and about 5" in diameter. Sprinkle with a pinch of salt. Cook for two minutes on each side until cooked through.

I like to toast the buns in the pan with some of the fat from the burgers, and serve with butter lettuce, sliced white onions, and sliced vinegar pickles (like cornichons).

# crispy cornflake chicken

**MAKES 8 PIECES** | LF | V | GF

Here's a delicous gluten-free crispy chicken. Marinating in a lactose-free "buttermilk" adds an extra layer of flavor.

## INGREDIENTS

**FOR MARINADE:**

2 cups almond milk

Juice and zest of 1 lemon

1 tablespoon salt

3 cloves garlic, crushed

Ground black pepper

**FOR COATING:**

3 cups corn flakes cereal

1 tablespoon paprika

2 teaspoons dried minced onion

2 teaspoons garlic powder

1 tablespoon dried sage

1 tablespoon thyme

1 tablespoon rosemary

1 teaspoon salt

## PREPARATION

Combine marinade ingredients in a baking dish and marinate chicken for 40 minutes, or up to 4 hours.

Preheat oven to 350°F (180°C). While chicken is marinating, combine all coating ingredients in a large food processor and pulse until everything is the consistency of bread crumbs. Spread crumbs onto large plate.

Brush a large parchment-lined baking sheet with olive oil or melted butter. With tongs, take chicken pieces out of marinade and dredge in crumb mixture. Place on baking sheet. When all chicken pieces are coated, brush or spray with oil or butter and bake until chicken is cooked through and crispy. Turn over each piece halfway through cooking time. Cooking time is about 35 minutes for boneless pieces or 1 hour for bone-in pieces. If chicken is browning too quickly, lightly tent with foil and remove for last 5 minutes of baking to crisp.

# seafood paella

**SERVES 6–8** | LF | GF
*Adapted from* La Tienda

This can be made in a 15" frying pan or two 10–12" pans if you don't have a paella pan. If your pan is smaller, it is important to use two pans so the rice doesn't end up mushy. It is also important to make sure you season as you go so that the rice ends up fully seasoned all the way through. Try not to stir once the rice has boiled, otherwise the rice sticks together.

When cleaning shellfish it is important to discard those that stay open when you tap them and those that have cracked shells. You can either add the shellfish to the rice in stages (as the clams take longer to open than mussels) or you can cook the shellfish separately (see instructions at the end of the recipe). Once they are cooked, discard any that did not fully open.

## INGREDIENTS

5 cups of fish or clam broth, plus an extra cup to add if there is no liquid left in pan after 15 minutes of cooking

2 teaspoons saffron

4 slices bacon, sliced into small pieces

6 tablespoons olive oil

1 red onion, diced

6 scallions, sliced green, tops reserved for garnish

1 red bell pepper, diced

8 cloves garlic, grated

2 large tomatoes, chopped

1 tablespoon fresh thyme, minced

2 teaspoons smoked paprika

2 cups paella rice such as Bomba of Valencia

1 dozen small clams (such as littlenecks), scrubbed

2 dozen mussels, scrubbed and beards removed

1 dozen large prawns, cleaned

2 tablespoons parsley

2 lemons cut into wedges

## PREPARATION

Heat broth in pot with saffron for 10 minutes. Cook bacon in 15" paella pan over medium heat until brown around edges. Remove 2 tablespoons of bacon and reserve for garnish. Add oil and cook onion, scallions, and bell pepper over medium heat for about 10 minutes until soft and slightly golden. Add garlic and cook for last few minutes. You'll want most of the moisture to cook out so they don't make the rice mushy, so feel free to cook for a few extra minutes if they seem wet. Season lightly with salt.

Add tomatoes, thyme, and paprika then cook for 10 minutes until tomatoes break down to form a sauce. Add salt to taste. Sprinkle rice over cooked tomatoes and toast for 3 minutes. While rice is toasting bring broth to a boil. Once boiling, pour over toasted rice and tomato mixture. Keep mixture boiling, stirring occasionally for 3 minutes. After this point you will not be stirring, so make sure it is seasoned to your liking.

Lower heat to point where rice is slowly simmering. You want it to bubble gently throughout but not be boiling. Simmer for about 15 minutes until it is no longer swimming in liquid. There will still be liquid in the pan but it will start to firm up. If there is no liquid left add additional cup of broth.

*Recipe continued on next page.*

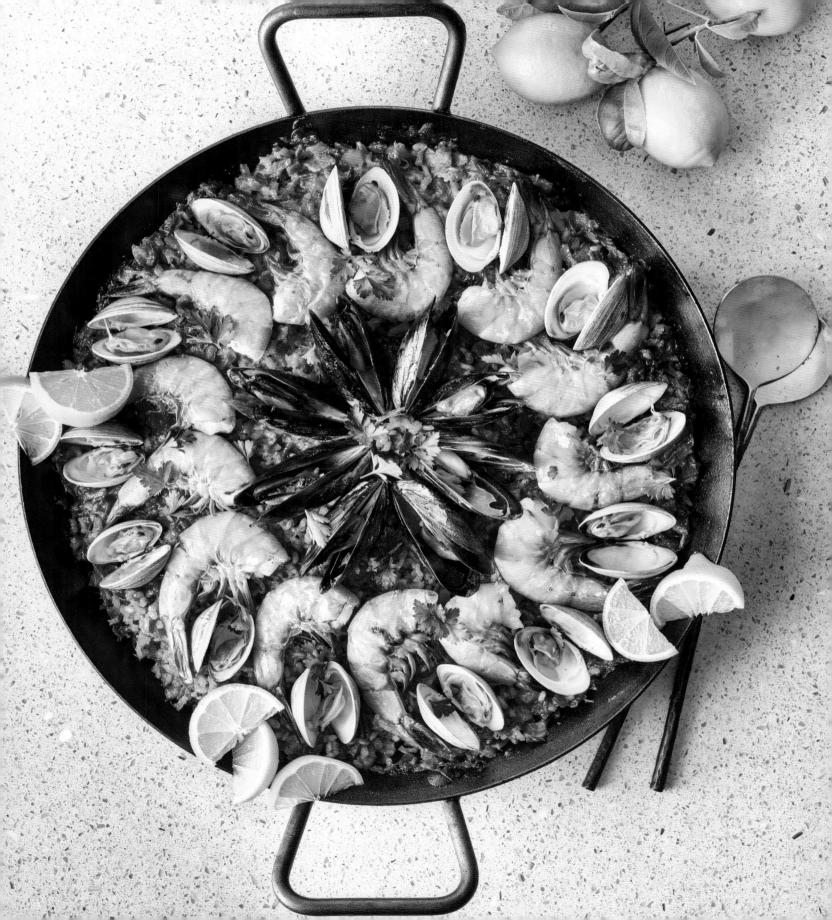

# seafood paella *cont.*

Add clams pressed into rice facing upwards and cover with foil for 12 minutes. After 12 minutes, gently lift foil and add mussels. Cover with foil and cook for 4 minutes. Lift foil up and add shrimp, then cook for an additional 5 minutes.

Cover pan tightly with foil and turn up heat to medium-high for 4 minutes to form crust on bottom of pan. Turn off heat and allow to steam, covered for 15 minutes more. Uncover and check rice for doneness. Rice should be tender, shrimp cooked through, and shellfish open at this point. If not, turn heat on high for another minute, cover and let sit for an additional 5 minutes. Garnish with parsley, reserved scallion tops, bacon, and lemon wedges.

**TO COOK SHELLFISH SEPARATELY:**
If you wish to cook clams and mussels on their own, you can simmer them in the broth until they open and set aside while rice cooks. Mussels will open after 4–6 minutes of cooking, clams after 8–10. Reserve broth to add to rice.

Follow instructions above for cooking tomatoes and rice. After initial 15 minutes of cooking rice, cover rice mixture with foil and cook for 20 minutes, adding raw shrimp and cooked shellfish for last 5 minutes of cooking.

Cover pan tightly with foil and turn heat up to medium-high for 4 minutes to form crust on bottom of pan.

Turn off heat and allow to steam, covered, for 15 minutes more. Uncover and check rice and shrimp for doneness. Rice should be tender, shrimp cooked through, and shellfish heated through. If not, turn heat on high for another minute, cover and let sit for an additional 5 minutes. Garnish with parsley, reserved scallion tops, bacon, and lemon wedges.

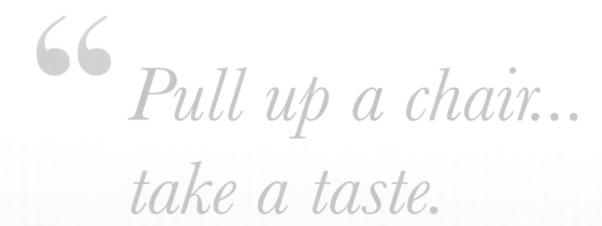

*"Pull up a chair... take a taste.*

# arctic char *with* succotash

**SERVES 6–8** | LF | GF

Here's a tasty dish, light and simple for a summer dinner.

## INGREDIENTS

2–2.5 pounds arctic char cut into 6 fillets

2 teaspoons sumac or zest of 1 lemon

1 large pinch salt

1 large pinch pepper

Olive oil

2 bell peppers, diced

1 bag frozen organic white corn
or fresh ears of corn shucked off the cob

¼ pound green beans, cut into ½" pieces

1 pint cherry tomatoes, quartered

1 bunch basil, chopped

## PREPARATION

Pat the artic char dry and dress with sumac, salt, and pepper. Grill on outdoor grill or indoors in a hot skillet and finish in the oven. If using outdoor grill, put the fish on foil and put the foil on the grill. For thicker fillets cook 6–7 minutes on each side, thinner fillets 3–4 minutes on each side.

If cooking indoors, preheat oven to 450°F (230°C). On the stovetop in an oven proof pan, sear fish with 1 tablespoon of olive oil, skin side down for 7 minutes. Transfer to oven and bake until fish is cooked through (5–7 minutes for thin fillets, 8–12 for thicker fillets).

While arctic char is cooking, cook bell peppers, corn, green beans, and tomatoes over high heat with a splash of olive oil and salt and pepper. Cook for 5 minutes until corn is cooked through. Remove from heat and toss with basil.

Serve arctic char, skin side up, on top of corn and tomato mixture.

*Come join us. Life is so endlessly delicious.* "

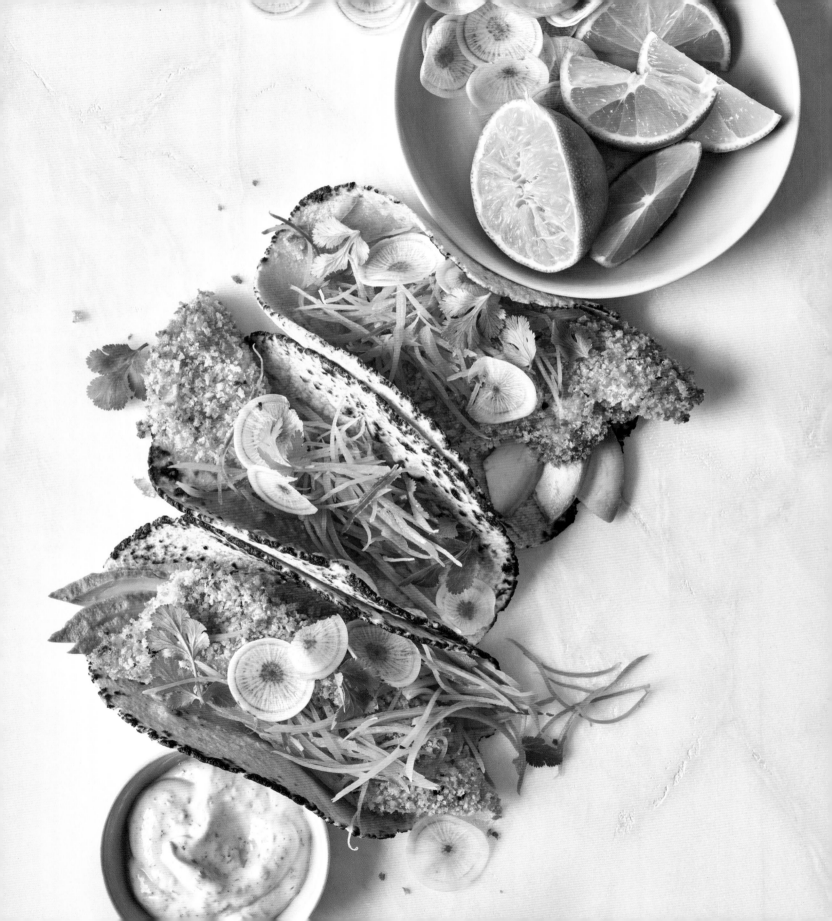

# fish tacos *with* creamy lime sauce

**SERVES 6–8** | LF

These can be made a couple of different ways. Sometimes in the summer when the weather is right for cooking outdoors, I'll skewer cleaned shrimp and toss them on the grill, cook them for a couple of minutes on each side, then toss them with garlic olive oil when they are done. Or, I'll use leftovers from the Whole Baked Branzino (p. 40) or the Fish Cooked in Parchment (p. 195) and top with the Creamy Lime Sauce (p. 91).

Or, you can make this crispy baked fish and have a healthier version of the fried fish tacos that are a family favorite. With some good corn tortillas, diced tomatoes and avocado, you have a healthy, kid-friendly dinner. Freezing the breaded fish pieces works beautifully to pop in the oven for when you are pressed for time. Great with Mango Salsa (p. 66), Carrot Jicama Slaw (p. 174), or Herb & Vinegar Infused Carrots (p. 128).

### INGREDIENTS

**CRISPY FISH:**

2 pounds of uncooked cod, cut into 1 × 3" strips

3 cups crispy bread crumbs

2 cups flour, seasoned with paprika, salt, and pepper

3 eggs, beaten

**CREAMY LIME SAUCE:**

¼ cup mayonnaise

½ avocado

½ bunch cilantro

Zest of ½ lime

Pinch smoked paprika

Lime juice, to taste

**GARNISH:**

Good quality corn tortillas

Avocado or guacamole

Diced tomatoes

### PREPARATION

Preheat oven to 425°F (220°C). Dredge each piece of fish in egg, then bread crumbs, and place on a parchment-lined sheet pan. Brush or spray with olive oil, cook for 5–6 minutes on each side, flip when bottom is crispy.

To make sauce, combine all ingredients in a small food processor and blend until creamy. Season to taste with lime juice, salt, and pepper

You can freeze the raw fish sticks on a sheet pan, and once they are frozen, put them in an airtight container. Pop them in the oven on a parchment-lined baking sheet for 7–10 minutes on each side until they are crispy and cooked through.

# berry lime granita

**MAKES 6 CUPS** | LF | V | GF

When summer berries are ripe and juicy, this bright and refreshing frozen dessert is a real sweet treat. Leftovers can be frozen and broken up again when you are ready to eat.

### INGREDIENTS

4 cups raspberries or blackberries

¾ cup caster sugar

Zest of 2 limes

¾ cup water

### PREPARATION

Combine all ingredients in food processor, process until smooth. Pour ingredients into a 9 × 13" baking dish. Place in the freezer for 3 hours. Every 30 minutes, use a fork to break up and scrape clumps of ice that begin to form.

# chocolate sauce

**MAKES 1 ½ CUPS** | V | GF

I love the Vegan Coconut Ice Cream (p. 95) with a big spoonful of warmed chocolate sauce, toasted sliced almonds, and a little crunchy salt on top. The coffee powder is optional but it does give the sauce a little something special—you won't notice the coffee, it just adds a little extra oomph. No one will believe this took you under 5 minutes to whip up.

### INGREDIENTS

1 cup high quality cocoa powder

1 cup sugar

½ cup water

1 tablespoon olive oil

1 teaspoon vanilla

½ teaspoon instant coffee or espresso granules

½ teaspoon salt

### PREPARATION

In a medium sized saucepan, sift cocoa powder over the top of the sugar. Add all other ingredients to pan and whisk over medium heat until it all comes together, about 3 minutes. It will thicken as it cools. Pour into a glass jar with lid. It will last for several months in the refrigerator.

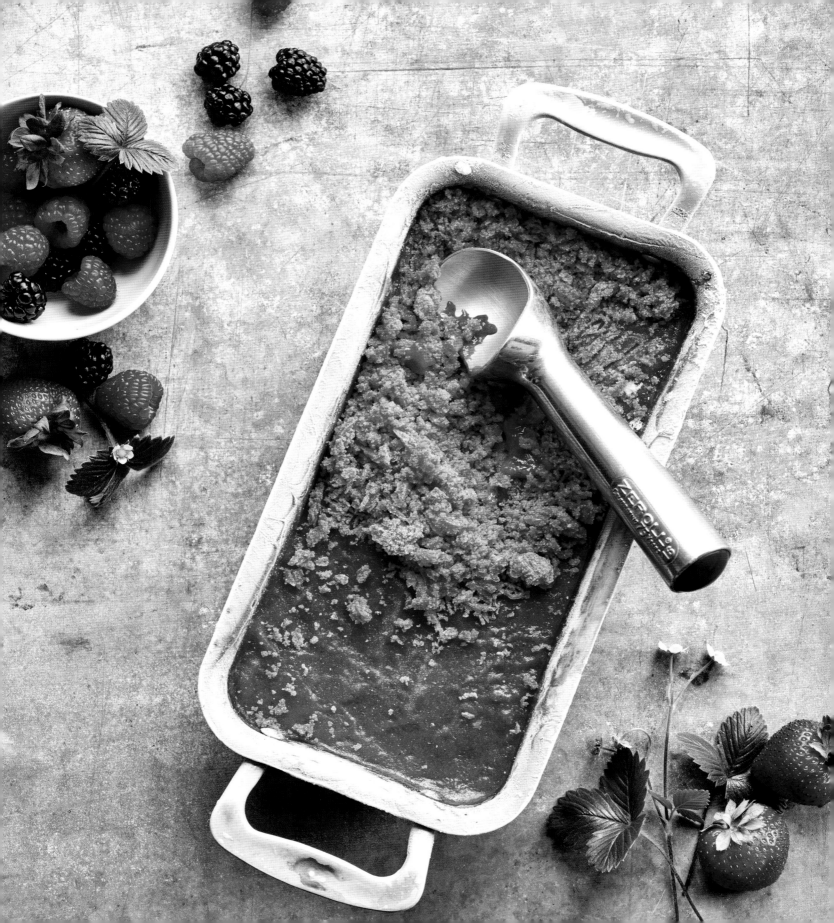

# flourless chocolate raspberry torte

**MAKES 1 (9") CAKE** | LF | V | GF

The base of this recipe is a luxurious flourless chocolate cake—already a fantastic cake, but I had a couple pints of berries calling my name. I made a quick jam and voilà, an easy, bright summer twist on this lush flourless chocolate cake. You can also add a little jam to your morning toast with ghee and crunchy salt.

## INGREDIENTS

**RASPBERRY JAM:**

2 cups berries

⅓ cup organic cane sugar

Juice of 1 lemon

**TORTE:**

¾ cup coconut oil

4 ounces bittersweet chocolate

4 ounces semisweet chocolate

2 tablespoons Raspberry Jam

½ teaspoon salt

## PREPARATION

To make the jam, mash berries, lemon juice, and sugar in a small saucepan with a potato masher until it turns into a raspberry sugar slush. Cook over low heat, stirring every few minutes until mixture thickens, about 15 minutes.

For cake, use parchment paper to line the bottom and sides of a greased 9" springform pan. Preheat oven to 350°F (180°C).

Melt the coconut oil with the chocolate, salt, and jam in the top of a double boiler and let cool.

While chocolate mixture is cooling, beat the egg yolks with the sugar until they become pale yellow. Mix the cooled coconut oil and chocolate mixture with the sugar and yolks. In a clean bowl, beat the egg whites until they are stiff but not dry. Gently fold into the chocolate mixture until just mixed together. It's okay if there are still a few white streaks in mixture, the important part is to make sure the egg whites stay nice and fluffy.

Gently pour batter into lined pan, smoothing top with spatula before putting in oven. Place a pan of water on the bottom shelf to help keep the torte from drying out. Bake batter in center of oven for 40–45 minutes, rotating pan after 20 minutes. When finished, the top will be puffed and slightly cracked. Remove from the oven and let cake rest for 15 minutes before unmolding and carefully peeling off the parchment paper. Carefully slide cake onto cake stand and let cool.

As the cake cools the center will fall, this is normal and makes for a nice center to fill with jam. When cooled, spread jam over the middle of the cake and dot edge with whole raspberries. Refrigerate for 1 hour until set.

# vegan coconut ice cream

**MAKES 2 CUPS** | V | GF
Adapted from Julia Turchen's *Small Victories*

This recipe rocks and will forever change my dessert game. It is hands down one of my favorite ice creams and pretty much anyone with any dietary issues can eat it. So easy and good, and there is no need for an ice cream maker—just a couple of empty ice cube trays, a freezer, and a few pantry items you probably already have on hand.

## INGREDIENTS

1 can (14 ounces) coconut milk

1 can (5.4 ounces) coconut cream

3 tablespoons maple syrup

1 teaspoon vanilla

2 pinches of salt

2 pinches nutmeg

## PREPARATION

Mix everything together in a medium-sized bowl. I like to do this in my big measuring cup since it is easier to pour from. It might take a little mushing to get the coconut cream and milk incorporated.

Pour into ice cube trays and let freeze overnight or for at least 4 hours. When frozen solid, dump them into a food processor. If the ice cubes don't pop right out, I find that running a fork around one edge of each cube helps to nudge them free. Pulse until cubes are broken into smaller pieces and then process for about 2 minutes, scraping edges a few times until it becomes smooth and creamy. If there are big chunks that won't break into pieces, let the mixture sit for a minute or two to soften and then keep processing.

Serve immediately or scoop into a glass jar and freeze for up to one week. If you are freezing it will need to sit for a few minutes until it becomes soft enough to scoop.

# spicy bloody mary

**MAKES 8 COCKTAILS** | LF | V | GF

You'll find a Bloody Mary cocktail on just about every brunch menu you'll ever see. It's a zesty, spicy, savory—and boozy—start to the day. If the alcohol isn't for you, omit it, it's just as tasty without it.

### INGREDIENTS

1 quart tomato juice

8 ounces lemon- or lime-infused vodka

2 tablespoons Old Bay Seasoning

2 tablespoon horseradish

Zest of 1 lemon

Juice of 2 lemons

1 tablespoon vegan Worcestershire sauce (Lord Sandy's is a good option), or coconut aminos

1 tablespoon brine from olives

1 tablespoon brine from capers

1 tablespoon rice vinegar

### GARNISHES:

Hot sauce, to taste

Salt, to taste

Freshly ground black pepper, to taste

Celery

Cucumber spears

Lime

Large caper berries

Olives

Radishes

Bacon

### PREPARATION

Mix together all ingredients. Season to taste with hot sauce and pepper.

If serving in a pitcher, stir vodka into mix and serve in glasses of ice and condiments. If making drinks to order, shake 1 cup of mix with 1–2 ounces of vodka and pour over ice.

Slide two olives, a radish, and a caper berry onto a toothpick. Prepare a toothpick for each glass.

Garnish each glass with celery stick, cucumber spear, lime, and toothpick garnishes.

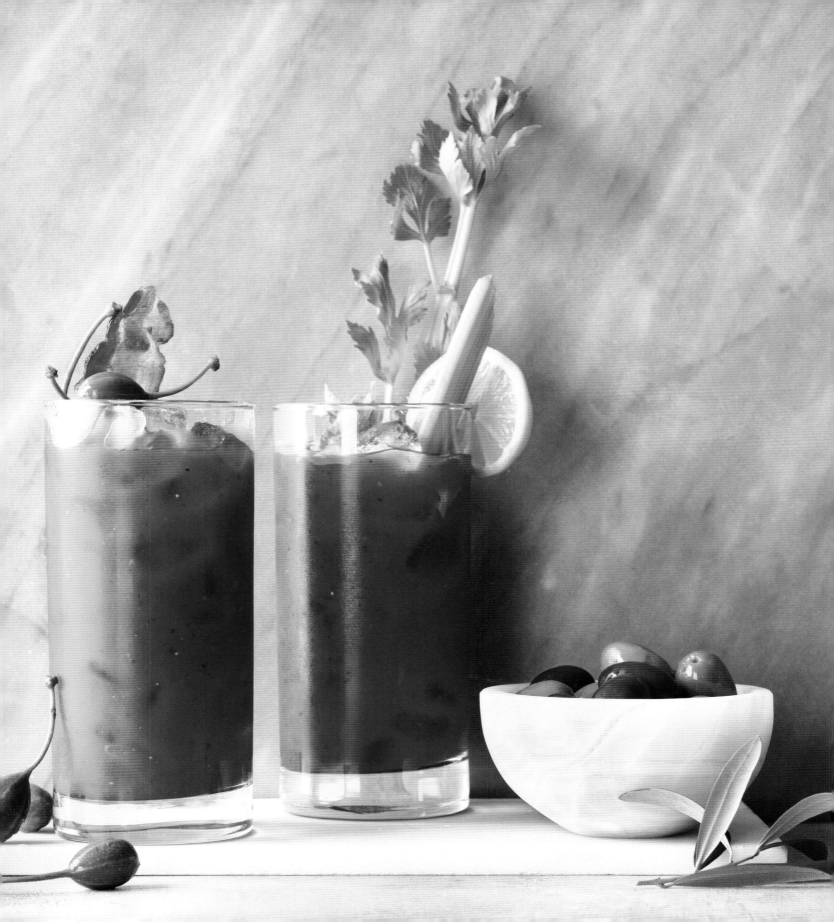

# strawberry cucumber refresher

**MAKES 1 COCKTAIL** | LF | V | GF

Summer sunsets call for a refreshing cocktail. Although there are many to choose from, this recipe is destined to be a favorite. The cucumber balances the sweetness and the strawberries and lime bring the tangy fruit goodness.

### INGREDIENTS

2 strawberries

4 sliced cucumbers, ½" thick

1 tablespoon caster sugar

Juice of ½ lime

2 ounces water

2 ounces vodka

### PREPARATION

Muddle strawberries and cucumber with sugar in bottom of shaker. Add lime, water, vodka, and ice. Shake, strain and serve.

# boozy blackberry granita

**MAKES 8 COCKTAILS** | LF | V | GF

This is a tart and refreshing summertime cocktail.

### INGREDIENTS

1 pint blackberries

Juice of 4 lemons

Zest of 2 lemons

3 tablespoons caster sugar + more to taste

3½ cups water

8–16 ounces vodka

### GARNISH:

Lemon slices dipped in sugar

Blackberries

### PREPARATION

Combine all ingredients except for vodka in a food processor, process until smooth. Pour ingredients into a 9 × 13" baking dish. Place in the freezer for 3 hours. Every 30 minutes, use a fork to break up and scrape clumps of ice that begin to form.

Scoop granita into glass and pour 1–2 ounces of vodka over the top and stir. Garnish with a sugared lemon slice and a blackberry.

# lemon verbena tea

**MAKES 1 QUART** | LF | V | GF

Lemony and bright, this is one of my favorite iced teas. It's best if you can find fresh leaves at the farmers market, but dried leaves from a health food store will do. Soothing for the nerves and stomach, and it has anti-inflammatory properties.

### INGREDIENTS

4 or 5 fresh lemon verbena sprigs, or 2 tablespoons dried leaves

1 quart boiling water

### PREPARATION

Pour boiling water over leaves and let steep for 5–15 minutes depending on how strong you like your tea. Strain and refrigerate for up to 3 days.

## Lemon Verbena

THE FRESH, CITRUS-MEETS-FLORAL SCENT WAS WHAT FIRST ELEVATED THE STATUS OF THIS RATHER UNREMARKABLE-LOOKING PERENNIAL SHRUB.

It is a noted favorite scent of women both real and fictional. Called out as the favorite scent of the mother of Laura Ingalls Wilder and the mother of Scarlett O'Hara, its essential oil is still used in the perfume industry today. It's also prized for its soothing effect on digestion and its anti-inflammatory properties, which are a result of its high levels of luteolin.

Pizza isn't just a meal, it's a food group unto itself. A SIBO diagnosis often leaves you feeling as if you have to give up everyday indulgences like pizza. We say—no way. We shall not be denied the chewy, cheesy satisfaction of pizza. A few tweaks, several trials later, and we brought these little slices of heaven back into our microbiome-balanced diets.

# PIZZA

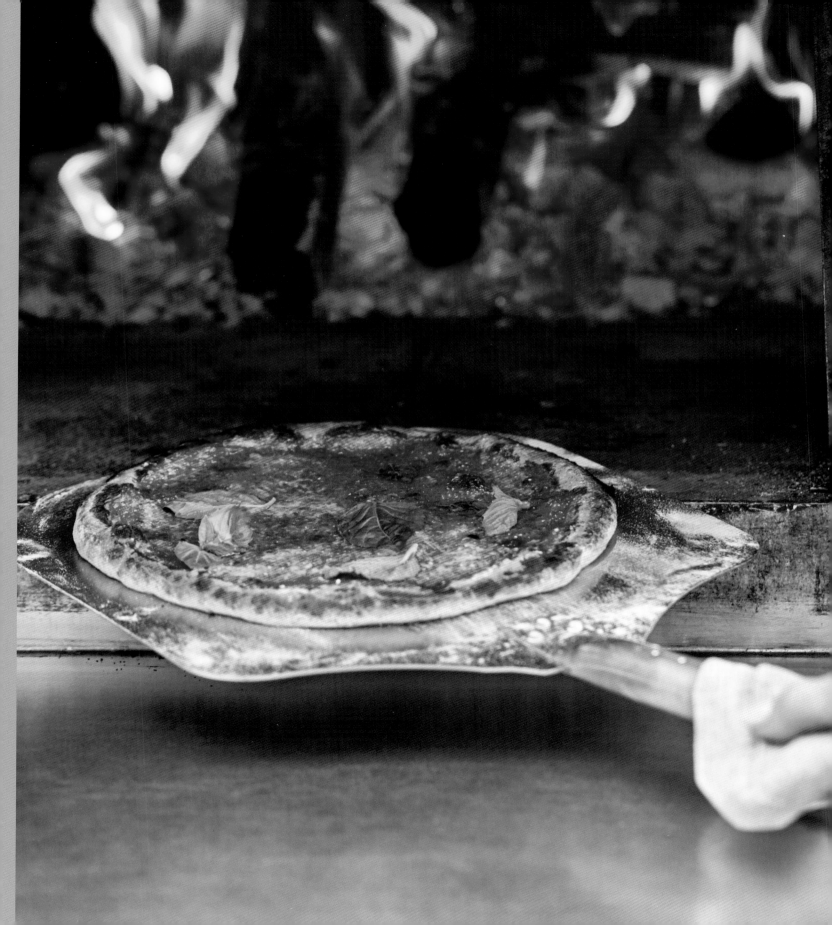

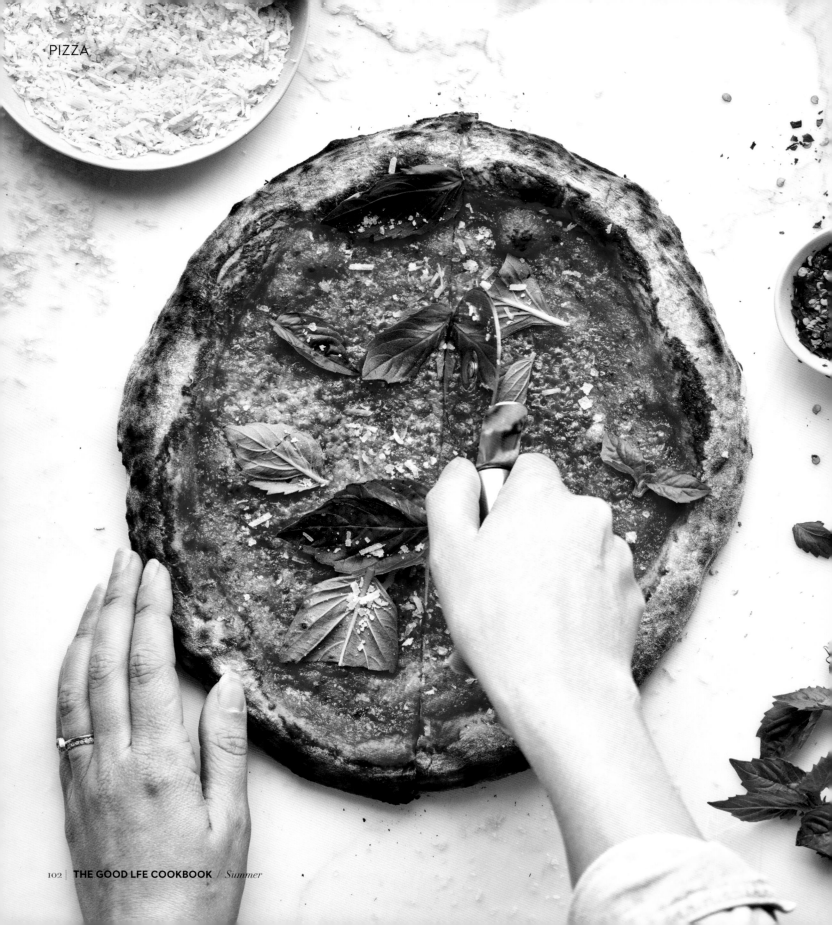

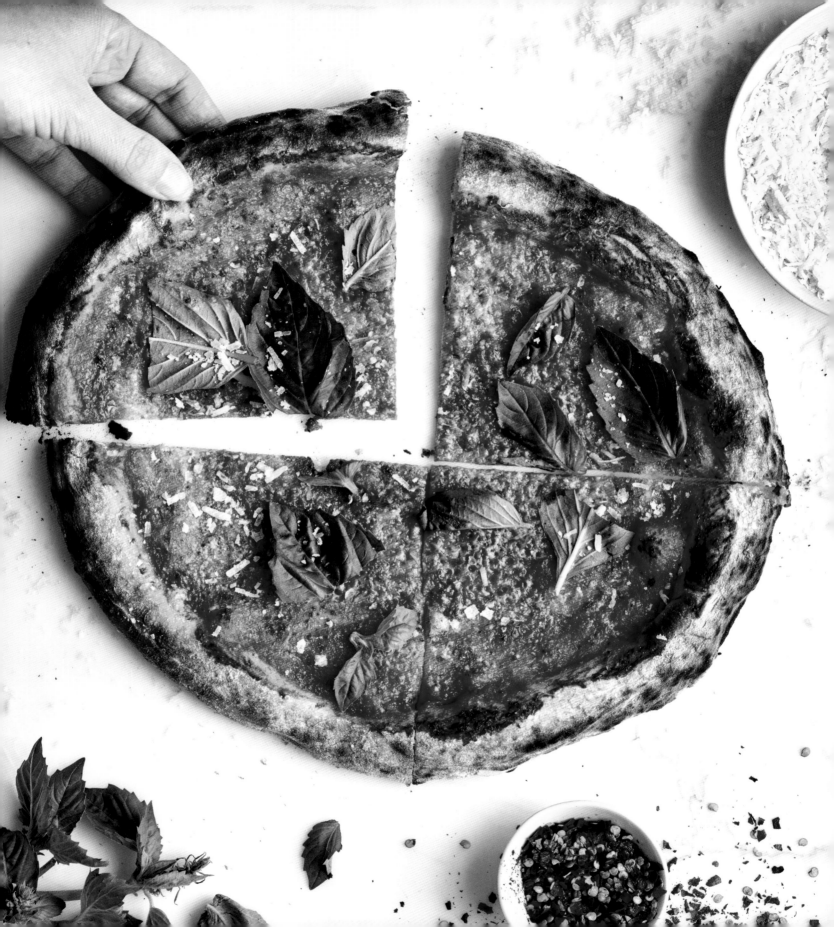

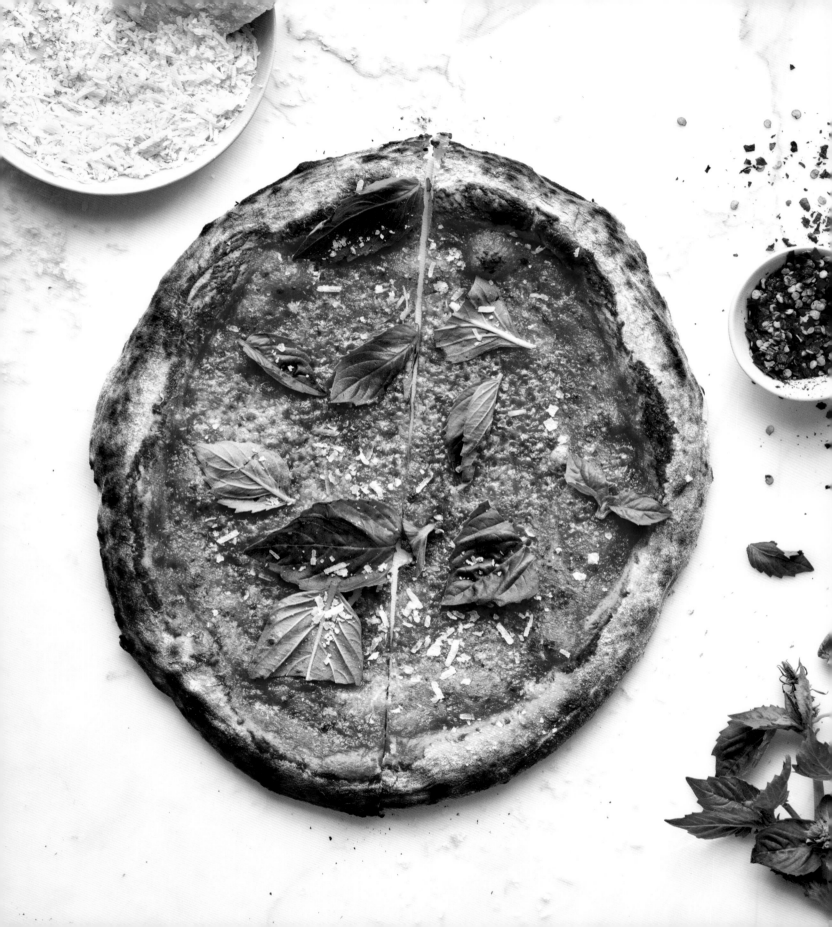

# pizza dough

**MAKES 4 (12") PIZZAS** | LF | V

This pizza dough is super easy to make, can be made up to 3 days ahead of time, and makes a classic Italian style dough. I find it easier to work with than store bought dough and just as good as any pizza I can get delivered.

## INGREDIENTS

1 pack active dry yeast

1½ cup warm water

Large pinch sugar

2½ cup all purpose flour + ½–1 cup for kneading

1 tablespoon salt

2 tablespoons oil

## PREPARATION

Mix yeast, warm water, and large pinch of sugar together in a small bowl. Let sit while you measure out other ingredients. It should create a slight layer of foam as it sits. This means the yeast is alive. If there is no foam and doesn't smell yeasty it means the yeast is no longer alive and you should start with a new packet of yeast.

In a large bowl mix flour and salt. Mound flour in the middle of bowl. Add oil to yeast-water mixture and pour around edges of flour mound. With a fork, gradually incorporate flour into water until it is fully mixed. Mixture will probably be quite sticky at this point.

Liberally flour counter surface or large sheet pan and scrape dough onto floured surface. Dust top of dough with ½ cup of flour and with floured hands begin kneading dough, adding flour until it just loses its stickiness. You may need to add up to 1 cup of flour but make sure to add gradually, as too much flour can make the dough too dry. This should take about 2 minutes. Overworking the dough will make it tough so knead only until there are no large lumps.

Divide dough into 4 equal pieces and roll into balls. Grease 4 small bowls, cups, or plastic containers then put one dough ball into each container and cover with plastic wrap. This dough can be made up to 3 days ahead of time and improves each day. If you are using dough right away, let sit in warm place until doubled in size about 1 hour.

If you are making dough ahead of time, you can let it slowly rise in the refrigerator, pushing dough down each day to make sure it doesn't escape the container.

# gruyère & parmesan pizza margherita

**MAKES 2 (12") PIZZAS** | LF | V

This is a lactose-free alternative to the classic pizza margherita. The pro tips for making pizza with a crisp golden crust in a home oven are to let the oven preheat for a good 30 minutes before baking, then allow it to reheat for a few minutes between baking when making multiple pizzas and don't overdue the toppings.

## INGREDIENTS

2 tablespoons olive oil

2 homemade pizza doughs

½ cup pizza sauce

½ cup grated Parmesan cheese

½ cup grated Gruyère

10 basil leaves, torn into pieces

## PREPARATION

Preheat oven to 500°F (260°C). Spread 1 tablespoon of olive oil onto a large sheet pan. Press dough into a 6" round on oiled sheet pan. Flip dough over so oiled side is up and continue stretching dough until it is a 12" round and ⅛" thick.

Spread ¼ cup of sauce over dough with the back of a large spoon. You should still be able to see dough through sauce. Top with ¼ cup of Parmesan and ¼ cup of Gruyère.

Bake for 10–12 minutes until crust is golden, use a spatula to lift up edge of pizza and check to make sure the bottom is also golden.

Top with torn basil before cutting and serving.

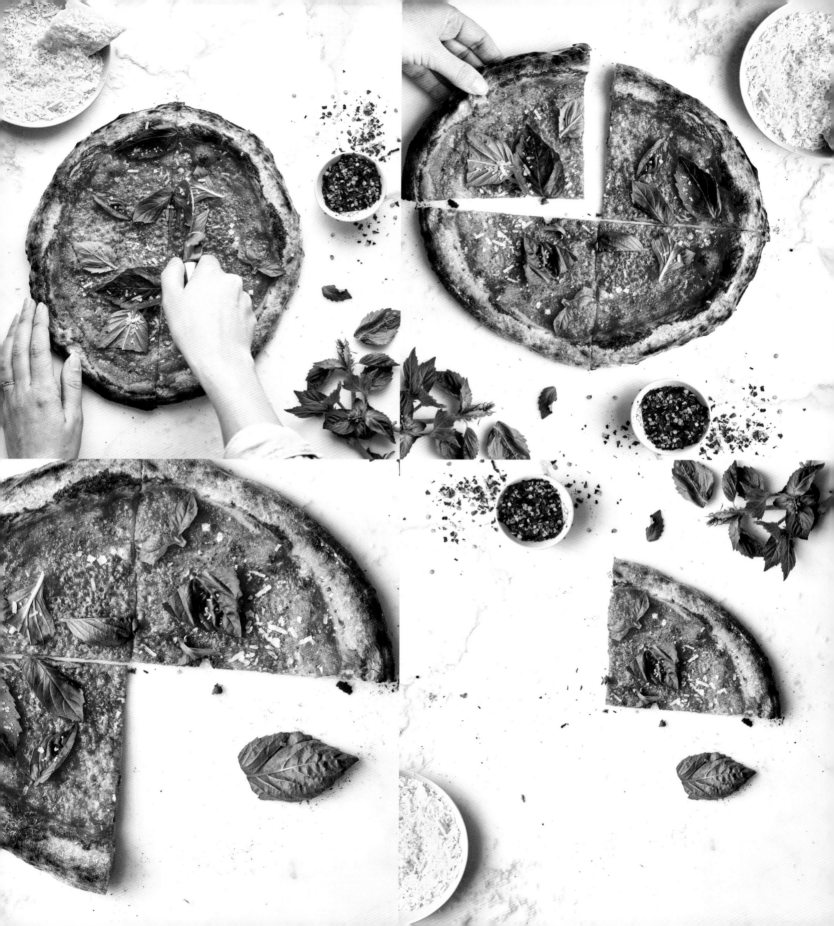

# pizza sauce

**MAKES 1 CUP** | LF | V | GF

Because the sauce will be cooked on the pizza while baking, there is no need to do anything other than add a little garlic, olive oil, and salt to either our homemade Simple Summertime Tomato Sauce (p. 79) or to a jar of high quality tomato sauce. We like the Mutti Passata that comes in a jar. One cup of sauce is about enough for 3–4 small pizzas or an extra large focaccia pizza.

### INGREDIENTS

1 cup tomato sauce

3 garlic cloves, grated on microplane

1 tablespoon olive oil

Salt to taste

1 sprig fresh oregano, chopped (optional)

### PREPARATION

Put everything in a jar and shake.

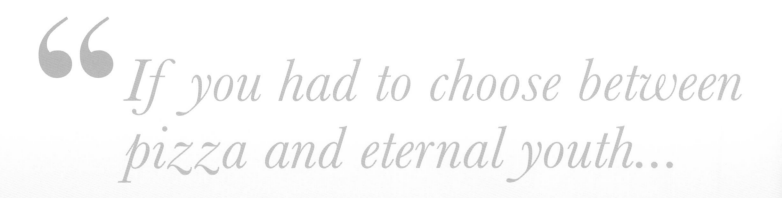

"*If you had to choose between pizza and eternal youth...*

# zucchini & lemon zest flatbread

**MAKES 2 (12 × 8") FLATBREADS** | LF | V

Here's a light springtime appetizer or a lunch with grilled vegetables. Make sure to slice your zucchini as thinly as possible so you don't end up with a soggy crust.

## INGREDIENTS

1 pizza dough

3 tablespoons garlic-infused olive oil

1 zucchini, cut into long ribbons with vegetable peeler

Lemon juice

Zest of 1 lemon

2 tablespoons thyme, minced

1 cup Parmesan cheese, shaved with vegetable peeler

Small handful of basil, chiffonaded

## PREPARATION

Preheat oven to 475°F (245°C). Press one ball of pizza dough into a ¼" thick rectangle on a greased sheet pan. Spread olive oil over the dough and sprinkle a pinch of salt. Bake for 6 minutes.

Toss zucchini with a light drizzle of olive oil, squeeze of lemon, thyme, lemon zest, salt and pepper.

Remove dough from oven and top with half of the Parmesan cheese. Lay zucchini over top of Parmesan and sprinkle with remaining cheese. Return to oven and bake another 5 minutes. Remove from oven and top with crunchy large flake salt and basil.

*...which toppings would you get on your pizza?* "

# wild mushroom *with* caramelized onions *&* gruyère flatbread

**MAKES TWO (12 × 8") FLATBREADS** | LF | V | GF

Who doesn't love pizza? This version gives you crispy edges, sweet onions, and plenty of gooey SIBO-friendly cheese. Thank goodness for Gruyère.

## INGREDIENTS

2 homemade pizza doughs

2 tablespoons olive oil

2 yellow onions, sliced

½ pound mixed wild mushrooms, sliced (shiitakes, oysters, chanterelles, and/or cremini)

1 tablespoon thyme, chopped

1 tablespoon parsley, chopped

1 teaspoons red wine vinegar

3 garlic cloves, minced

Large handful of parsley, minced

1 cup Gruyère cheese, grated

Zest of 1 lemon

Salt and ground black pepper, to taste

## PREPARATION

In a large sauté pan set over medium-low heat, heat 1 tablespoon olive oil. Add the onions and a generous pinch of salt and cook for 30–45 minutes, stirring regularly, until the onions are caramelized. If onions are browning too quickly, lower heat. Add another tablespoon olive oil, mushrooms, thyme, and another generous pinch of salt and pepper. Cook 10–12 minutes, until mushrooms are very tender.

Turn heat up to medium-high and add red wine vinegar, garlic, and parsley. Scrape bottom of pan, loosening brown bits and stir for 3 minutes more until vinegar has evaporated and edges of mushrooms start to brown. Season to taste. Mushrooms often need quite a bit of salt.

The mushroom mixture will store well in the refrigerator and can be made a few days ahead of time.

### FOR FLATBREADS:

Preheat oven to 475°F (245°C). Press one ball of pizza dough into a ⅛" thick rectangle on a greased sheet pan, about 12" wide and 8" long. Drizzle a bit of olive oil over the dough and sprinkle with a pinch of salt. Bake for 6 minutes.

Remove dough from oven and top with onions and mushrooms, followed by the crumbled Gruyère and remaining thyme. Return to oven and bake another 5 minutes. Remove from oven and top with minced parsley, lemon zest, crunchy large flake salt, and shaved truffle.

Using a pizza cutter, slice the flatbreads into 2 × 3" slices.

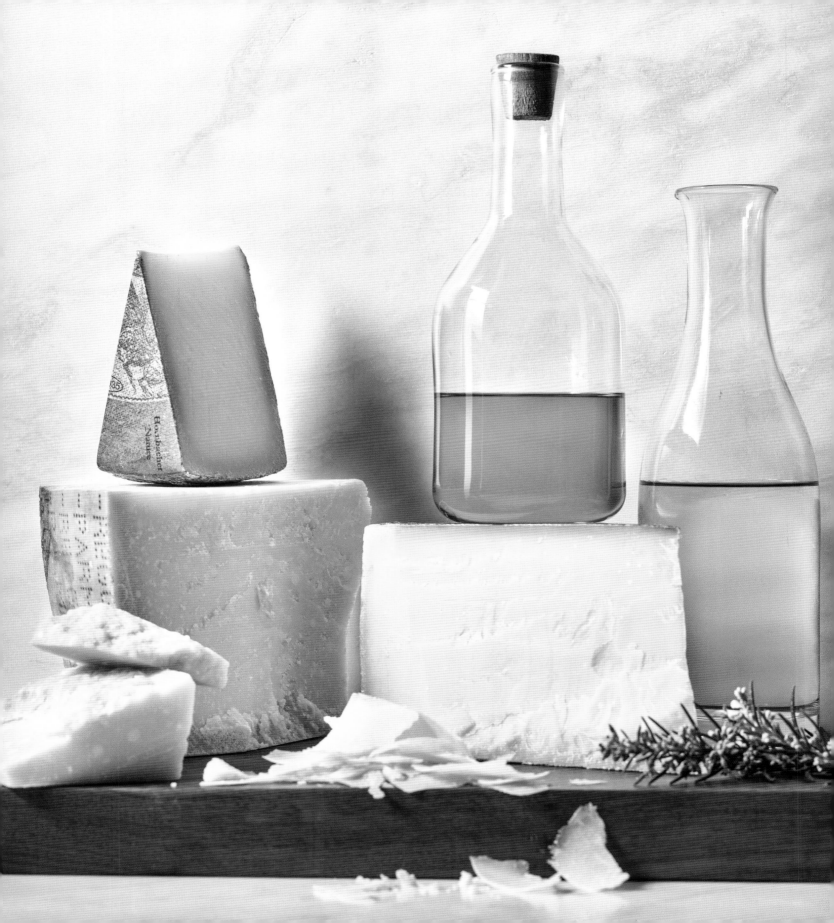

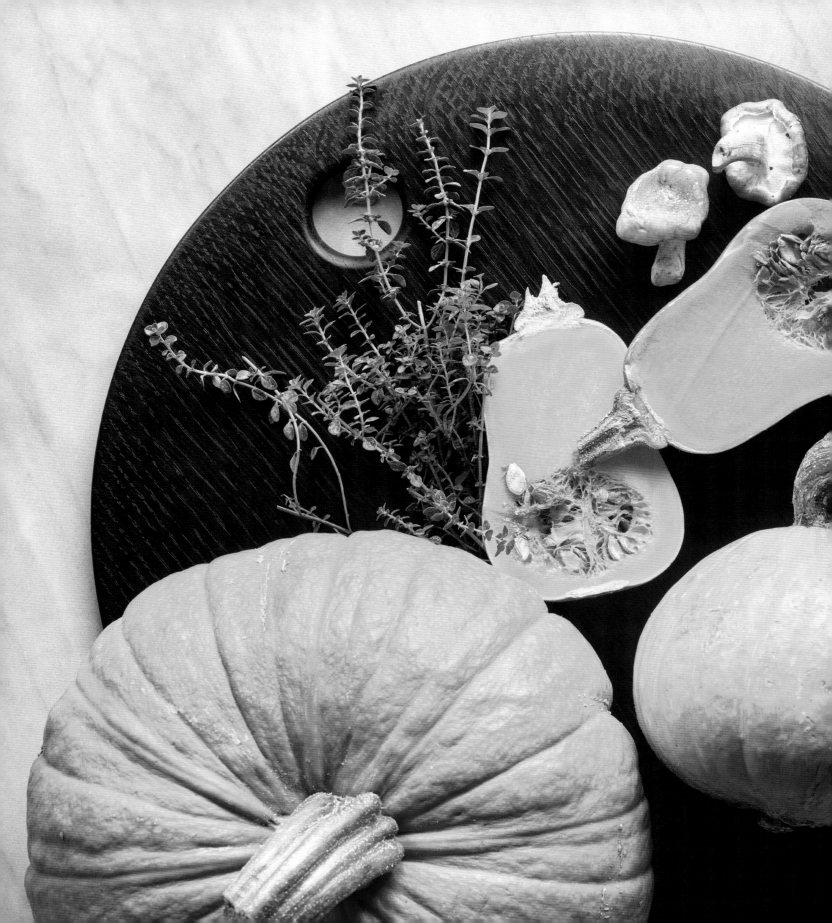

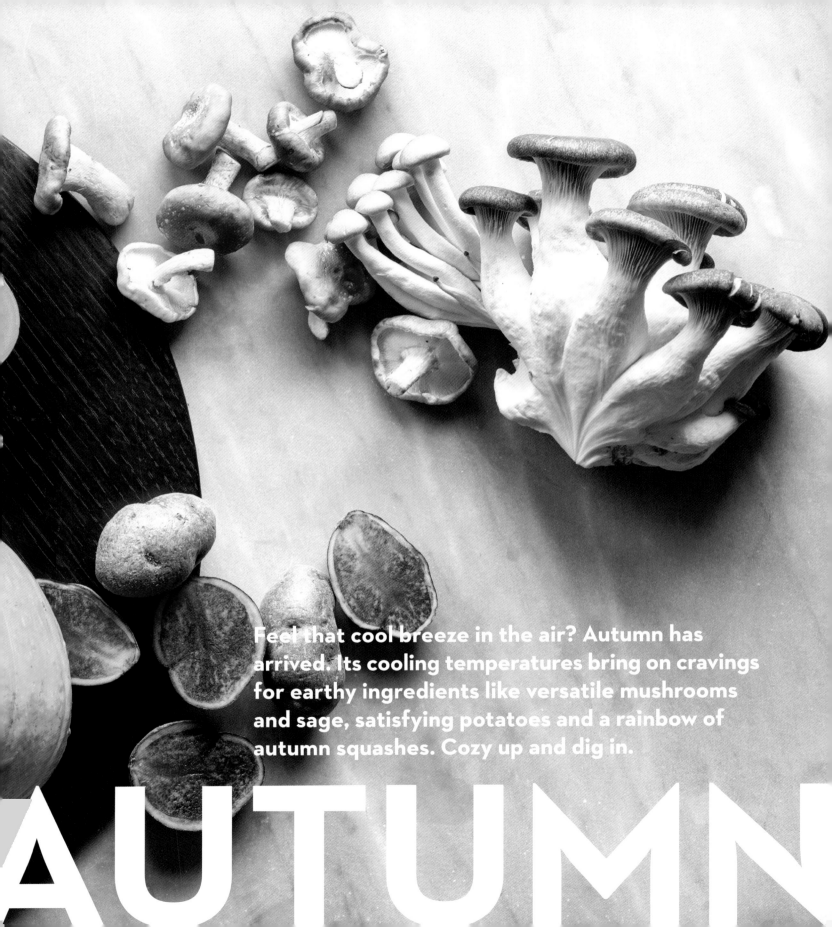

Feel that cool breeze in the air? Autumn has arrived. Its cooling temperatures bring on cravings for earthy ingredients like versatile mushrooms and sage, satisfying potatoes and a rainbow of autumn squashes. Cozy up and dig in.

# AUTUMN

Autumn's arrival is heralded by a cool that we feel in our bodies and spirit. It's a time to slow down, settle in, and enjoy the chill.

Relaxing our pace does wonders for our digestion. And what's good for our gut is great for our microbiome. We have a season's worth of autumnal recipes that make the most of the warm spices and earthy vegetables that are good for our health and a treat for the senses. Tuck in and enjoy!

# sweet potato & bacon sheet pan hash

**MAKES 3 CUPS** | LF | GF

This brunch recipe can be scaled up or down very easily—it's half a sweet potato and two pieces of bacon per person with some onion thrown in. If you'd like to have eggs, you can add one or two per person and bake for an additional 8–10 minutes until the yolks are as runny or firm as you like.

## INGREDIENTS

3 sweet potatoes, cut into ½" cubes

6 preservative-free, organic bacon slices, cut into ½" rectangles

1 onion or leek, cut into a large dice

1 tablespoon thyme, minced

## PREPARATION

Preheat oven to 400°F (200°C). Toss all ingredients on a large parchment-lined sheet pan, making sure the bacon is evenly distributed throughout. Bake for 30 minutes or until potatoes are browned and bacon is crispy. Stir once during cooking.

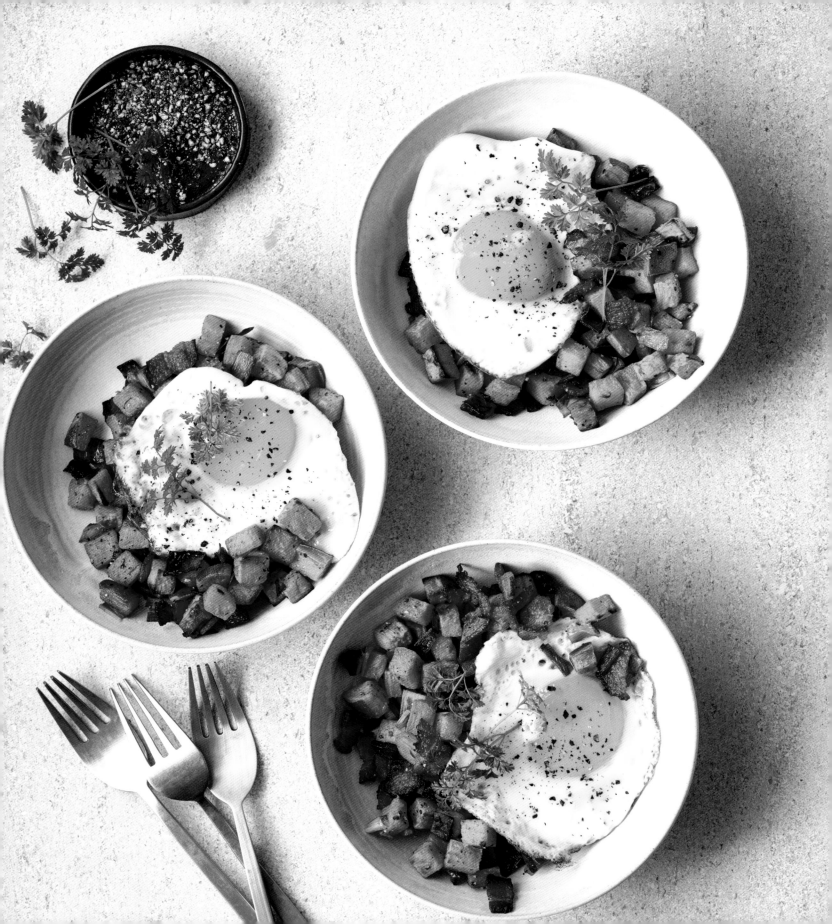

# coconut rice porridge

**MAKES 3 ½ CUPS** | LF | V | GF

If you're craving a warm and nourishing breakfast, give this delicious rice porridge a try. The cardamom and vanilla with the maple syrup create a sweet and fragrant blend. Feel free to add berries or a crunchy topping to this creamy bowl of goodness.

**INGREDIENTS**

1 can (15 ounces) of coconut milk

1 cup jasmine rice

2 tablespoons maple syrup

1 tablespoon vanilla extract

½ teaspoon cinnamon

½ teaspoon cardamom

¼ teaspoon nutmeg

½ teaspoon salt

1 ½ cup almond milk + more if needed

1 cup sesame granola or toasted and sliced almonds

Handful of blueberries, strawberries, or banana slices

**PREPARATION**

Bring coconut milk to a boil in a medium-sized saucepan. Add rice, boil for 5 minutes, cover and simmer over low heat for 20 minutes. Add maple syrup, vanilla, spices, salt, and almond milk. Stir and cook for another 10 minutes, uncovered over low heat. Remove from heat, cover, and let sit for 5 minutes.

To serve, top with nuts and yogurt. Pour almond milk over the top if you like it a little creamier.

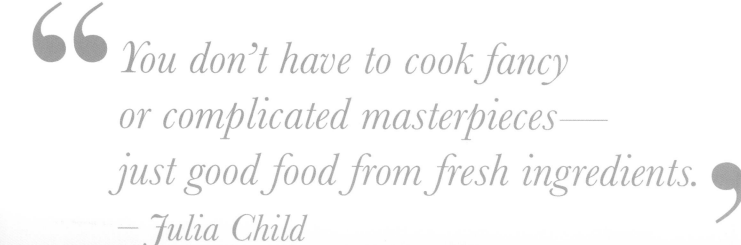

*"You don't have to cook fancy or complicated masterpieces— just good food from fresh ingredients."*
*— Julia Child*

# autumn delicata frittata

**MAKES 1 (12") FRITTATA** | LF | V | GF

Roasted delicata squash is tender and earthy, and an easy alternative to the potato found in many frittata recipes. The caramelized onions add a layer of flavor and pair deliciously with the savory squash.

### INGREDIENTS

2 Roasted Delicata Slices (p. 132)

6 onions, caramelized for 1½ hours until reduced to 1 cup

1½ teaspoons salt

Handful of parsley, chopped

1 tablespoon thyme, chopped

1 tablespoon ghee or butter

1 cup Gruyère cheese, grated

1 bunch chives, finely chopped

12 eggs + 1 can (5.4 ounces) coconut cream + 1¼ teaspoon of salt blended in blender or with hand blender until frothy

### PREPARATION

On the stove over low heat, layer half of the roasted delicata in an appealing pattern in the bottom of 12" cast iron pan that is liberally oiled with ghee (or butter). Sprinkle with half of the herbs and salt. Top with caramelized onions, 1 cup of cheese, remaining herbs, and egg mixture. Lay remaining squash in a pattern on top of egg mixture and finish with the rest of the cheese.

Cook over medium heat on stove until edges of frittata start to set.

Bake at 400°F (200°C) for 15 minutes until middle of frittata is set and a knife inserted in the center comes out clean. It will continue to firm up over next 10 minutes.

# breakfast burrito

**MAKES 1 BURRITO** | LF | V

Start the day with this warm and delicious breakfast burrito and you'll be fueled for hours. The toasted exterior paired with the juicy and flavorful interior is a combination everyone will enjoy.

### INGREDIENTS

1 flour tortilla

4 tablespoons aged Cheddar cheese

Large handful of baby spinach

2 Perfect Fried Eggs (p. 10), cooked for an additional few minutes until yolks are lightly cooked

¼ avocado, mashed or two tablespoons guacamole (optional)

5 cherry tomatoes, diced and tossed with a squeeze of lime and salt

Butter or olive oil

Salt and ground black pepper, to taste

### PREPARATION

Place tortilla in a frying pan over medium heat.* Toast on one side for three minutes until warm. Flip and add cheese to tortilla. When cheese is melted, remove tortilla from pan and add a small amount of olive oil. Add spinach with a pinch of salt and sauté for 2 minutes until wilted. Spoon onto a tortilla. Prepare eggs and place on top of spinach. Add avocado or guacamole and top with tomatoes. Wrap tightly into a burrito.

*If making multiple burritos, warm tortillas topped with cheese on a parchment-lined sheet pan at 350°F (180°C) for 5 minutes while preparing other ingredients.

# parmesan crisps

**MAKES 16 (1") CRISPS** | LF | V | GF

My favorite part of anything topped with cheese and baked are the bits of cheese that fall onto the pan and turn into little crispy morsels. So, for all the other crispy cheese lovers out there—this one's for you. Serve with Carrot Romesco (p. 18), as a topping for soups, or on their own as a crispy nibble.

### INGREDIENTS

½ cup Parmesan cheese, finely grated

### PREPARATION

Preheat oven to 350°F (180°C). On a parchment-lined baking sheet place heaping teaspoons of cheese 2" apart. Lightly pat down tops of cheese mounds. Bake for 15 minutes until cheese is bubbly and golden and edges are a little darker than the rest. Let cool. When firm to the touch, place on paper towel and chill. They can be stored for a week in an airtight container in the refrigerator. If they lose their crispness you can re-crisp them in a hot oven for a few minutes.

# garlic knots

**MAKES 12 SMALL KNOTS** | LF | V

A half recipe of Pizza Dough (p. 105) makes 12 small knots. Dipping them in the garlic sauce both before and after baking gives you a nice combination of crunchy garlic and gooey garlic, so be sure to do both steps.

### INGREDIENTS

1 stick butter or ½ cup olive oil or mix of both

10 garlic cloves, minced

Small handful oregano, minced

Small handful parsley, minced

½ recipe Pizza Dough (p. 105)

Parmesan cheese, grated

### PREPARATION

Preheat oven to 400°F (200°C). Over low heat, melt butter or oil in small saucepan with oregano, parsley, and garlic. If using unsalted butter or olive oil, season with salt to taste.

Divide risen pizza dough into 12 balls. Roll each ball into a strip about 3" long and tie in a knot. Dip into melted garlic oil. Place a on parchment-lined baking sheet. Bake 10–15 minutes until golden brown. Cooking garlic oil/butter over low heat, continue poaching in garlic oil/butter while knots bake. After knots come out of the oven, spoon leftover garlic oil/butter over tops and sprinkle with Parmesan cheese or crunchy salt.

# spinach parmesan pinwheels

**MAKES 8 PINWHEELS** | LF | V

Easier than you might think, these tasty wheels make a great after school snack or appetizer for gatherings. Each bite is a harmony of flavors.

## INGREDIENTS

Olive oil

2 large cloves garlic, minced

2 bunches spinach, washed, stems removed and chopped

½ recipe Pizza Dough (p. 105)

1 cup Parmesan cheese, finely grated

Salt and ground black pepper, to taste

## PREPARATION

Preheat oven to 350°F (180°C). In a sauté pan over medium heat, heat oil, add spinach and garlic evenly throughout, and cook until spinach is wilted. Let cook for a few minutes longer if needed to make sure most of the water from spinach has evaporated.

Once pizza dough has risen, spread on a large, well oiled sheet pan into a large rectangle about ⅛" thick. Brush with olive oil, sprinkle ¾ cup cheese evenly on dough, and season with pepper. Spread spinach over cheese and tightly roll into a long jelly roll log. Cut into rounds that are 2" wide and lay on parchment, cut side up, flatten into a 1" thick round. Sprinkle with remaining cheese. Bake for 30 minutes until cooked through and light golden brown.

These are also quite tasty without cheese. If not using cheese, sprinkle 2 tablespoons nutritional yeast along with a couple pinches of salt over your dough rectangle brushed with olive oil before adding spinach.

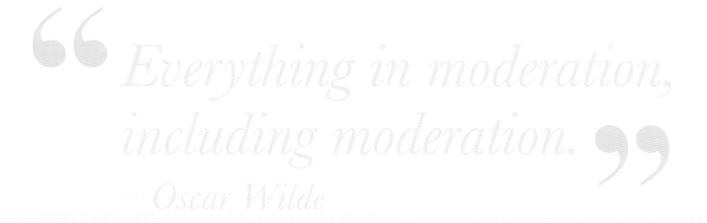

*" Everything in moderation, including moderation. "*
*— Oscar Wilde*

# veggie dumplings

**MAKES 2 DOZEN DUMPLINGS** | LF | V

A brunch favorite, we keep them simple with a little touch of Everything Spice on top. The filling can be spooned or piped in. If you are making the dumplings ahead of time, keep the filling separate until the day you are serving them, this will keep filling from becoming runny.

## INGREDIENTS

½ pound mushrooms, finely chopped

3 carrots, grated

3" piece of ginger, finely grated

1 bunch scallions, finely chopped

1 bunch spinach, finely chopped

2 cloves garlic, finely grated

2 tablespoons coconut aminos

Juice of ½ lime

½ teaspoon sesame oil + more to taste

1 tablespoon salt

2 tablespoons avocado oil or other neutral oil

3 tablespoons sesame seeds, toasted

3 tablespoons panko bread crumbs

1 package dumpling wrappers

1 scallion, thinly sliced for garnish

Everything Spice (optional)

## PREPARATION

Heat oil in a large skillet over high heat, sauté mushrooms, carrots, and ginger with a large pinch of salt and pepper until mushrooms are lightly browned. Add scallions, spinach, garlic, coconut aminos, lime juice, and cook until spinach is wilted and moisture has evaporated. Stir in sesame seeds and season to taste.

To assemble dumplings, place wrappers under a damp paper towel. Fill a small bowl with water for wetting edges of wrappers. Fill the middle of wrapper with one teaspoon of filling, wet edges with water and fold wrapper in half, sealing edges and pressing out any air. Place finished dumplings on parchment-lined sheet pan.

To steam, line a bamboo steamer with lettuce or cabbage leaves and place steamer over pot of boiling water. Steam until wrappers become translucent and filling is hot, about 5–8 minutes.

If you don't have a bamboo steamer, you can improvise by steaming on lettuce or cabbage leaves in a small amount of water in a large skillet with a lid.

Garnish with sliced scallions and serve alongside Asian Dipping Sauce (p. 125).

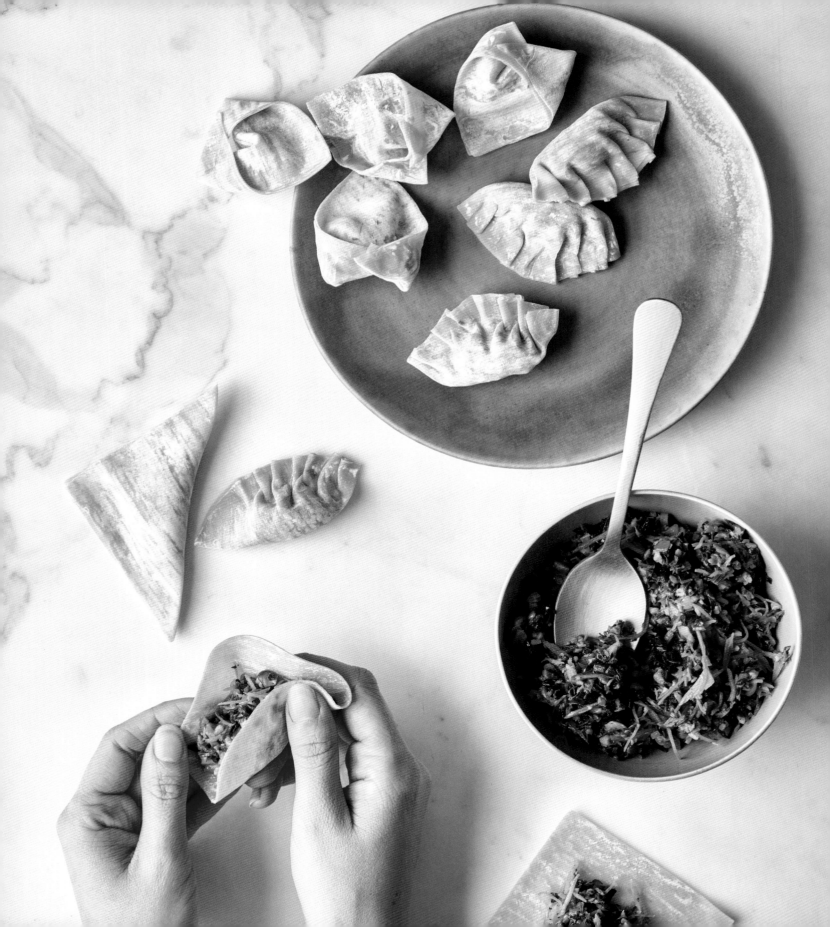

# cheese dip

**MAKES 2 CUPS** | LF | V | GF

For something with a texture that emulates the smooth consistency of a Velveeta-based cheese dip, look no further than the Super Gooey Scientific Mac & Cheese sauce (p. 187). Below are some ideas for additions you can make if you want to spice it up.

### INGREDIENTS

⅓ recipe Super Gooey Scientific Mac & Cheese sauce (p. 187)

### PREPARATION

**SPINACH AND GARLIC**

Wilt 1 bunch of spinach with 2 cloves of garlic in sauté pan over medium heat until water has evaporated. Add to cheese sauce and pulse with hand blender until spinach is incorporated (to your liking). You can stir in chopped water chestnuts to add a little crunch. Serve with baguette slices.

**SALSA CON QUESO**

For a Tex-Mex dip, omit the nutmeg and add a small can of roasted mild green chilies and a pinch of cumin to the sauce. Serve with tortilla chips.

# cashew sour cream

**MAKES 1 ½ CUPS** | LF | V | GF

Here's a rich, tangy, and tasty replacement for the typical dairy-based sour cream. Start with raw cashews, and after a long soak, blend with remaining ingredients for a simple and smooth dip or dollop for your favorite chili.

### INGREDIENTS

1½ cup cashews, soaked in water overnight, drained, and rinsed

¼ cup water + more if needed to make creamy

1 tablespoon lemon juice

2 teaspoons rice vinegar

¼ teaspoon salt

### PREPARATION

Place all ingredients into the bowl of the food processor or use a high-powered blender like a Vitamix or bullet-style blender. Blend until creamy. In the food processor, blending will take a little more time, so continue for 4–5 minutes, scraping the bowl every couple of minutes. If you find the cream to be too grainy, add water by the tablespoon until it is the desired consistency. Season to taste with lemon juice and salt.

# asian dipping sauce

**MAKES ½ CUP** | LF | V | GF

This is a versatile sauce that can be used with dumplings, steamed vegetables, Asian-style salads, or poured over fish before steaming. Coconut aminos make a great substitute for soy sauce and add a little sweetness. Feel free to add a few drops of toasted sesame oil if you are in the mood for something with a little more depth.

**INGREDIENTS**

3 tablespoons low sodium soy sauce or coconut aminos

3 tablespoons rice vinegar

Juice and zest of ½ lime

1 teaspoon chili sauce

1 teaspoon ginger, finely grated

½ shallot, finely grated

1 garlic clove, finely grated

**PREPARATION**

Mix all ingredients together and let sit for 10 minutes before serving. To use as a salad dressing, add 1–2 tablespoons neutral oil like avocado or sunflower.

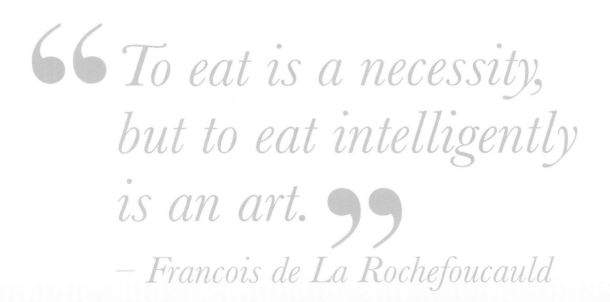

*To eat is a necessity, but to eat intelligently is an art.*

*— Francois de La Rochefoucauld*

# caramelized onion dip

**MAKES 1 ½ CUPS** | LF | V | GF

This is a dairy-free rendition of the classic onion dip. Take it to a party and no one will ever know it's dairy-free. Make it as a present for your vegan friends. Feel free to spice it up if you like it spicier. It's good with chips, toast, or French bread.

## INGREDIENTS

1 small yellow onion, diced

1 leek, cleaned and sliced thinly (you can use two onions if you don't have a leek)

1 recipe Cashew Sour Cream (p. 124)

Splash white wine (optional)

1 small bunch chives or 3 green onions, finely chopped

Handful parsley, finely chopped

1 teaspoon paprika

1 teaspoon garlic powder

1 teaspoon onion powder

1 teaspoon dill

Pinch cayenne

Lemon juice, salt and pepper, to taste

## PREPARATION

Brown onions and leeks in olive oil for 5–10 minutes over medium-high heat with a pinch of salt. Add a splash of white wine and scrape brown bits off bottom of pan. Turn heat to low and caramelize onions for 1 hour until soft and golden and reduced to about one-third of the volume of the raw onions.

Add caramelized onions and all other ingredients to the Cashew Sour Cream. Season to taste with salt, lemon juice, and pepper.

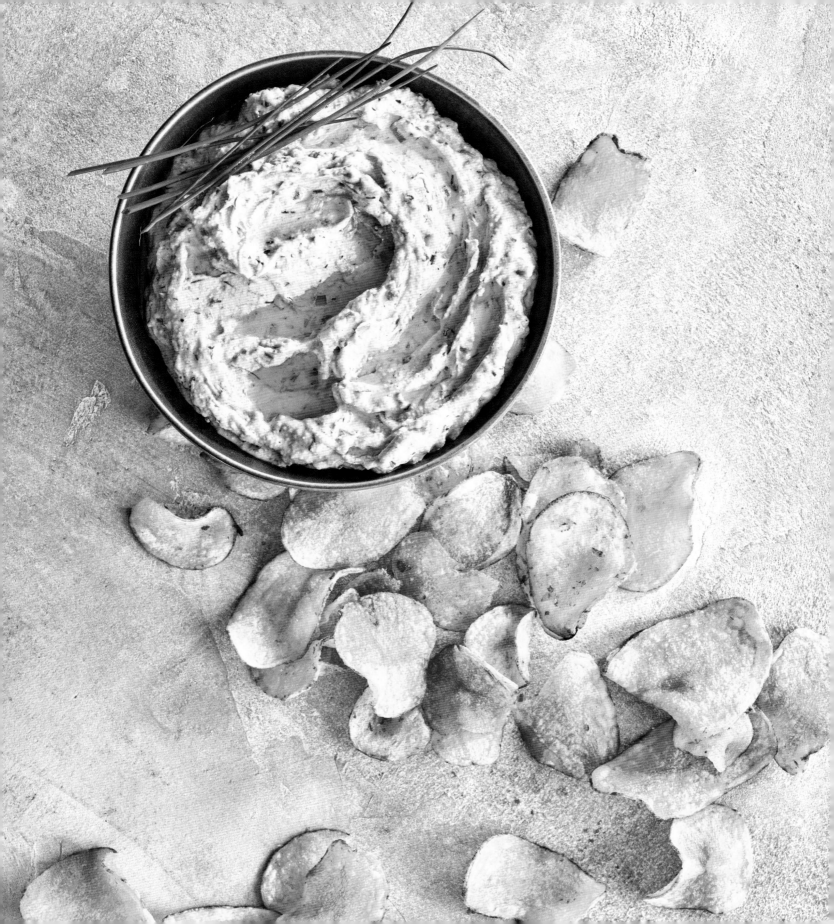

# herb & vinegar infused carrots

**MAKES 1 PINT** | LF | V | GF

This is a little ode to those giant, awesome jars of spicy pickled vegetables that are displayed on taqueria counters in San Francisco and Los Angeles. A big forkful adds a fresh crunchy tang to tacos and are great on sandwiches or just straight out of the jar as a snack. This mellow version omits jalapeños but feel free to add the seeded and quartered peppers if you like it spicy.

### INGREDIENTS

3 carrots, cut in half lengthwise and sliced on a bias

½ red onion, thinly sliced

3 garlic cloves, peeled

½ cup water

¾ cup apple cider vinegar

1 tablespoon sugar

1 teaspoon sea salt

2 bay leaves

¼ teaspoon red pepper flakes

### PREPARATION

Place vegetables in a 2 cup glass jar.

Heat the remaining ingredients in a small saucepan until simmering. Carefully pour hot liquid over vegetables and press down into pickling liquid. Add more water if needed to cover. Allow to marinate at least 1 hour before serving.

# pomegranate vinaigrette

**MAKES 1 CUP** | LF | V | GF

Similar to a balsamic vinaigrette, this one has a little bit of a fruity tang. Great on spinach salads or use it to marinate chicken before roasting.

### INGREDIENTS

3 tablespoons pomegranate molasses

3 tablespoons lemon juice

2 teaspoons caster sugar or maple syrup

1½ tablespoons Dijon mustard

½ cup olive oil

Salt and ground black pepper, to taste

### PREPARATION

Whisk all ingredients together in a bowl. Season to taste.

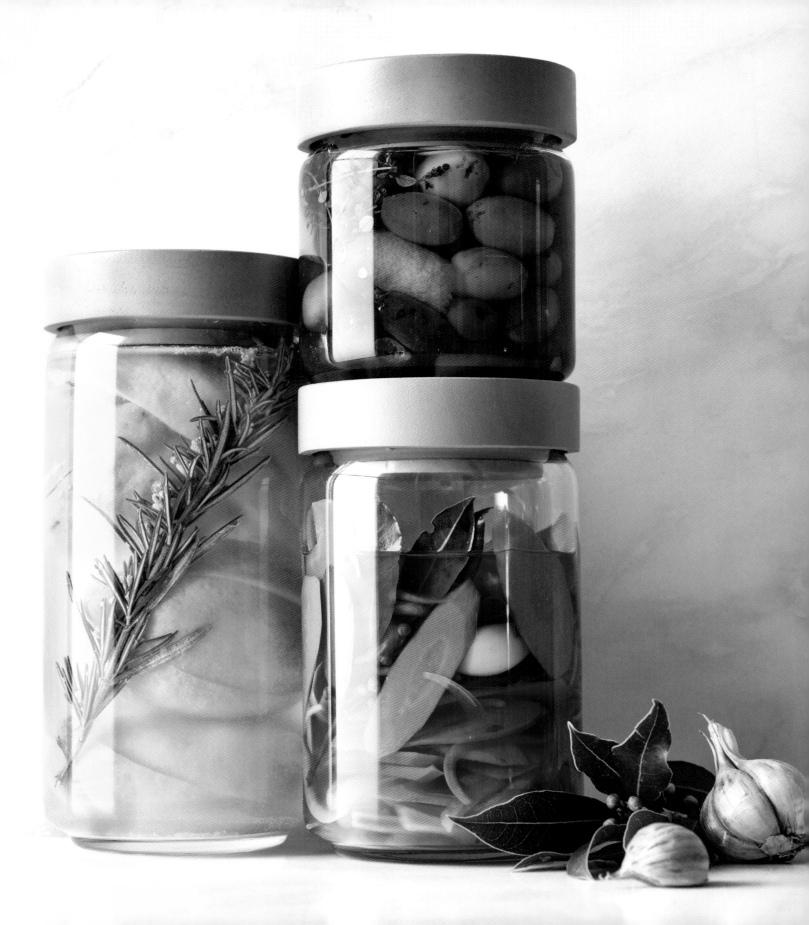

# butternut squash sage soup *with* cashew cream

**MAKES 2 QUARTS** | LF | V | GF

Simply put, this autumn in a bowl.

### INGREDIENTS

**SOUP:**

2 tablespoons olive oil

2 leeks, washed thoroughly, drained and chopped

20 sage leaves, chopped

1 large butternut squash, peeled, seeded, and cut into 1" cubes (about 6 cups)

3 garlic cloves, minced

3½ cups chicken broth (or vegetable broth for vegans)

¼ teaspoon ground black pepper

Generous pinch each of ground cardamom, cinnamon, cloves, nutmeg, and cayenne

Sea salt

1 recipe Cashew Sour Cream (p. 124)

**FRIED SAGE LEAF GARNISH:**

10 sage leaves

2 tablespoons olive oil

### PREPARATION

In a large pot, heat the olive oil over medium heat. Add leeks and sage along with a pinch of salt and sauté until tender, about 6 minutes.

Add butternut squash, spices, and two generous pinches of salt. Stir and cook until browned around edges. Add garlic and sauté until fragrant.

Add the broth, another generous pinch of salt, and black pepper. Bring to boil, reduce to simmer and cook, covered, until the squash is tender, about 30 minutes.

While squash is cooking, make the Cashew Sour Cream and set aside. Fry sage leaves in olive oil until crispy, about 3 minutes, then drain on paper towel.

Carefully, blend the soup in the pot with immersion blender until creamy adding half of the cashew cream and additional broth or water as necessary. If using a countertop blender, let soup cool for 20 minutes and blend in batches until creamy and return to the pot.

Season soup to taste with salt, pepper, and cayenne.

Serve soup topped with a dollop of cashew cream and fried sage leaves.

# creamy tomato soup

**MAKES 3 QUARTS** | LF | V | GF

My absolute favorite tomato sauce recipe is the lovely Marcella Hazen's version. It is as simple as can be—tomatoes, butter, and a quartered onion all simmered together to make magic. I have also made it with olive oil and it is a delicious vegan substitute. This soup is based on that sauce with potatoes and carrots to make it creamy, and honey to round out the acidity of the tomatoes. Add whatever herbs you have on hand—basil and dill are two of my favorites, but if there are others you prefer, go for it. Parmesan Crisps (p. 120) are awesome with this soup.

## INGREDIENTS

5 cups Simple Summertime Tomato Sauce (p. 79) or 2 large cans organic peeled and diced tomatoes

2 onions, peeled and quartered

3 carrots, cut into rough chunks

3 small potatoes

6 tablespoons butter or olive oil

1 teaspoon honey

Bunch of dill or basil, picked and roughly chopped

Salt and ground black pepper, to taste

## PREPARATION

Combine tomatoes, onions, carrots, potatoes, salt, and butter in large pot. Let simmer for 1 hour until all the vegetables are soft. Use a stick blender to blend until smooth. Add honey, salt and pepper to taste. Add herbs and blend for a few seconds more.

Miraculously, our digestion automatically shifts to make the most of the bounty of the season. In fall and winter when denser foods like gourds, tubers, and grains are filling our plates, our bodies automatically increase levels of amylase, a starch-digesting enzyme, and we also experience a boost in our overall digestive energy.

# roasted delicata slices *with* warm spices

**MAKES 6–8 SERVINGS** | LF | V | GF

Every time I make this I'm asked what the trick is for making this squash so tasty. Delicata squash is just that good all on it's own. All it needs is salt, olive oil, and an oven hot enough to get it nice and crisp. If the pan isn't too crowded, the squash will crisp on both sides without flipping it over. Or, if you are using a couple sheet pans and it's steaming rather than crisping, it's easy enough to flip the slices with a wide spatula and turn oven to broil for two minutes to make it crispy.

Dress it up for a dinner party with salsa verde and crunchy roasted squash seeds or just top with flaky salt. Usually half of a medium-sized squash per person is sufficient and will provide plenty to snack on before it makes it to the table. Depending on how hungry your guests are, you might have some leftovers.

Bonus snack: Pick the seeds out of the squash pith, roast with a little salt at 350°F (180°C) for 20 minutes or until they are toasty brown. Give them a stir and a shake halfway through.

## INGREDIENTS

3 squash, cut in ½, seeds removed, sliced into ¼" thick half moons

½ teaspoon of warm spices—cinnamon, coriander, garam masala, or ras el hanout in any preferred proportions to equal ½ teaspoon

Generous pour of olive oil

Salt

## PREPARATION

Preheat oven to 450°F (230°C). Toss everything in a big bowl and lay out on a single layer on a parchment-lined sheet pan. Bake for 20 minutes. If both sides are not browning, flip over and place under broiler for 3 minutes until edges are dark and bubbly.

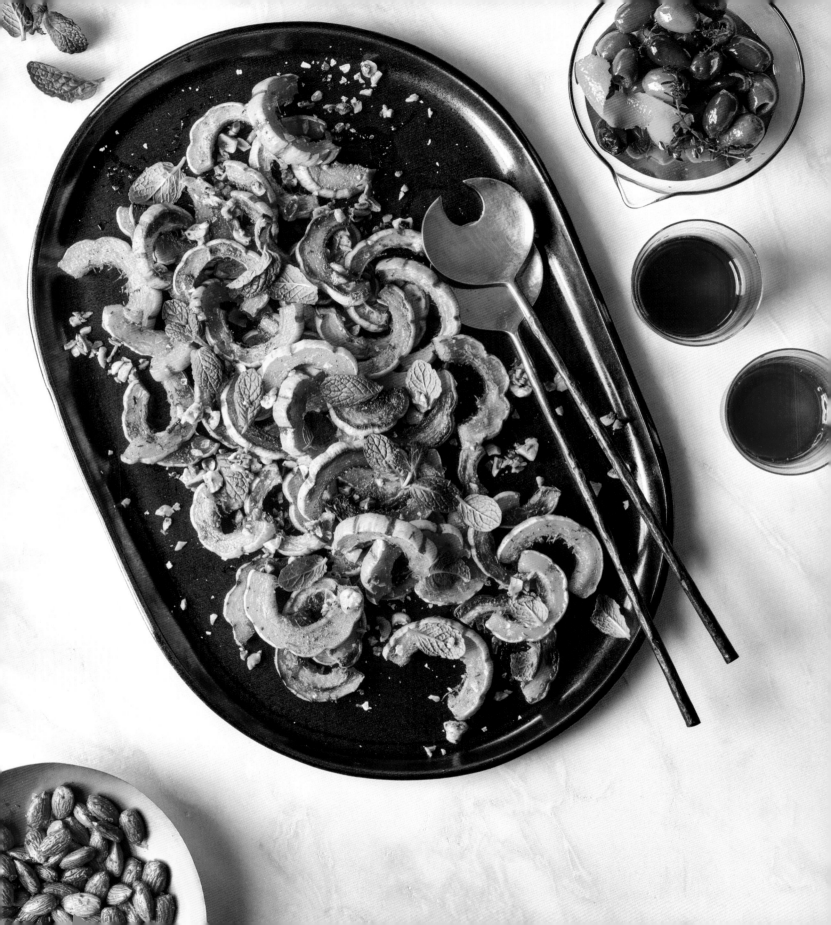

# creamy mashed potatoes

**MAKES 6 SERVINGS** | LF | V | GF

A basic, creamy mashed potato recipe that can be played with to your liking. We love the creaminess the cashew cream adds, and the olive oil can be replaced with butter or ghee; other options can be added based on what you are serving.

### INGREDIENTS

4 pounds Yukon Gold potatoes

¼ cup chicken broth (or vegetable broth for vegans) + more as needed

Salt

Ground white pepper

1 half recipe Cashew Sour Cream (p. 124)

⅓ cup olive oil

1 tablespoon nutritional yeast

### OPTIONAL ADDITIONS:

½ cup chopped chives

10 cloves roasted garlic

2 tablespoons chopped thyme

### PREPARATION

Cut potatoes in half and cover with cold water in a large pot. Starting the potatoes in cold water helps them to cook evenly all the way through. Heavily salt the water and bring to a boil over high heat. Lower heat to medium and cook 25–30 minutes, until potatoes can be easily pierced by a fork.

While potatoes are cooking, make the Cashew Sour Cream.

Warm broth in a small pot.

Drain potatoes and let them sit in pot over low heat to allow any excess moisture to evaporate. Slowly add olive oil and three large pinches salt while mashing, still over low heat. Add cashew cream, nutritional yeast, and gradually add stock, continue to mash until they are creamy and fluffy. Season to taste with salt and pepper.

# baked spaghetti squash

**MAKES 4–6 SERVINGS** | LF | V | GF

Cutting the squash into rings keeps the squash strands long to use in place of spaghetti. Great with pasta sauce or on their own tossed with garlic butter and herbs. If squash are on the smaller side go ahead and roast three.

### INGREDIENTS

2 spaghetti squash, washed

Olive oil

Salt

### PREPARATION

Preheat oven to 400°F (200°C). Cut ends off squash and cut into 1" rings. Scoop seeds out of each slice with a spoon. Place on parchment-lined sheet pan and lightly drizzle each side with olive oil and sprinkle with salt. Bake for 1 hour until tender. Scoop flesh out with a spoon, fluff with fork and season to taste.

# fluffy spanish rice *with* fried almonds

**MAKES 3 CUPS** | LF | V | GF

This is one of those side dishes that can pair with anything just by switching up the seasonings. When I make this as a side with something a little more French or Greek, I substitute the tomato paste for lemon juice and a long strip of lemon peel, and I trade the cilantro for a mix of parsley and thyme or oregano. If I'm making something more Middle Eastern, I skip the tomato paste and add a cinnamon stick and a ¼ teaspoon each of ground allspice and cloves while I'm toasting the rice.

## INGREDIENTS

**RICE:**

1 onion, finely diced

1 stalk celery, finely diced

2 tablespoons olive oil, ghee or chicken fat

1 cup rice

¼ teaspoon turmeric

1½ cup vegetable broth or chicken broth

1 tablespoon tomato paste

½ teaspoon salt

Bay leaf

**GARNISH:**

¼ cup slivered almonds

Two pinches ground coriander

Handful of cilantro, chopped

Salt and ground pepper, to taste

## PREPARATION

On stovetop, sauté onion and celery over medium heat for 10 minutes until brown around the edges. Add rice and toast about 5 minutes, adding a little more oil during toasting if rice sticks to the bottom of pan. Cook until rice is slightly golden and translucent, add garlic and turmeric for the last couple of minutes of toasting. Thoroughly toasting the rice will help make finished rice fluffy.

When rice is well toasted add broth, tomato paste, and salt then stir until tomato paste is dissolved. Bring to a rolling boil. Turn heat to low, cover and cook for 15 minutes. Remove from heat and let stand for 15 minutes more while covered. Fluff with fork. If still damp, leave in pot for 5 minutes more and fluff again. Season to taste.

While rice is resting, add two teaspoons of olive oil to a small frying pan over medium heat. Add almonds with a pinch of salt and a couple pinches of ground coriander and fry for 2–3 minutes until light golden brown.

Top finished rice with cilantro and fried almonds.

# yellow curry chicken

**SERVES 6–8** | LF | V | GF

This is a one-pot meal with meat and vegetables. Braising the chicken with its skin on gives it a nice crispy exterior with tender meat. Make sure to season as you go and add the green beans towards the end of cooking so they don't overcook. I like to serve this right out of the pan with jasmine rice.

## INGREDIENTS

1" piece of ginger, minced

3 garlic cloves, chopped

2 shallots, diced

1½ tablespoons yellow curry powder

¼ teaspoon smoked paprika

¼ teaspoon ground coriander

1 can (13.5 ounces) full fat coconut milk

1 can (5.4 ounces) coconut cream

½ cup broth or water

Juice of 2 limes

3 carrots, peeled and cut into 1" slices

4 potatoes, peeled and cut into 2" pieces

1 whole chicken, cut into 10 pieces (breasts cut in half)

⅓ pound green beans, ends trimmed and cut in half

¼ cup cilantro, minced (about 1 bunch)

½ teaspoon maple syrup

## PREPARATION

Preheat oven to 400°F (200°C). In a large oven-safe skillet or cast iron pan over medium heat, sauté ginger, garlic, shallots, curry powder, paprika, and coriander in a small amount of oil or ghee. When everything is toasted and fragrant, add coconut milk, coconut cream, and a ¼ cup broth or water and stir. Season to taste with lime juice, and salt and pepper. When coconut cream is melted and everything is combined, remove from heat. Add carrots and potatoes to pan.

Liberally season chicken pieces with salt and pepper and place, skin side up, on top of vegetables in coconut milk. Nestle chicken down into vegetables but make sure the skin is not submerged. Spoon coconut milk lightly over chicken pieces.

Bake for 45 minutes, gently lift up chicken with tongs and gently stir green beans into sauce. Place chicken back on top and bake for an additional 15 minutes until chicken and vegetables are cooked through and skin is a dark golden brown. Taste for seasonings and add lime juice, and salt and pepper if needed. Garnish with cilantro and serve with rice.

# SPICE IT UP

*Beyond adding taste, depth, flavor, and variety to foods without adding calories, research shows that herbs and spices contain a spectrum of health-promoting properties. They contain a high density of phytonutrients, vitamins, minerals, and antioxidants, often in levels much higher than found in fruits and vegetables. Some microbiome-aiding herb and spice standouts are:*

---

- **Ginger stimulates digestion, fights nausea, relieves bloating, and supports overall gut health.**

- **Turmeric is an excellent source of curcumin, a well researched anti-oxidant with evidence showing that it may reduce inflammation, boost immunity, and possibly even ease pain. In addition, it's believed to improve high blood pressure and high cholesterol, and it contains anti-cancer properties.**

- **Cinnamon and garlic both boast anti-inflammatory properties. Cinnamon is also anti-microbial and garlic helps boost our immune system.**

- **Oregano contains 4× the antioxidant power of blueberries. Antioxidants fight free-radical damage and inflammation linked to aging, cancer, and chronic diseases.**

- **Mint, sage, hibiscus, and nettles all deliver anti-inflammatory benefits— add them to boiling water for a warming tisane. Rosemary, thyme, basil, and chamomile add color and flavor to foods, and add anti-oxidants to your microbiome.**

# cast iron chicken *with* caper lemon croutons

**SERVES 6–8** | LF

This recipe calls for caper berries, which are the large capers with stems. You can substitute 2 tablespoons common capers if need be. Crisping the croutons in the pan with the chicken fat adds flavor and keeps them from getting soggy. An easy one-pan dinner for a weeknight yet impressive enough to serve for a dinner party.

When photographing this recipe for the cookbook, the chicken fat croutons were our favorite kitchen snack—pretty irresistible.

## INGREDIENTS

### MARINADE:

Zest of 1 lemon

½ cup lemon juice (about 3 lemons)

1 teaspoon salt

½ teaspoon ground black pepper

3 garlic cloves, minced

2 tablespoons caper berry brine

2 tablespoons maple syrup

1 tablespoon Dijon mustard

3 tablespoons olive oil

1 bunch each fresh thyme and oregano, chopped divided in half (reserve remaining half for croutons)

10 pieces bone-in, skin-on chicken (for example, 2 breasts, 4 thighs, 4 drumsticks)

### CROUTONS:

1 baguette, ripped into 2" cubes

1 jar (2 ounces) caper berries, stems removed, roughly chopped

Half of the chopped herbs

Olive oil, as needed

## PREPARATION

Combine all marinade ingredients in a shallow baking dish. Place chicken in baking dish, cover with plastic wrap and marinate for at least 2 hours and up to overnight, turning chicken over once or twice.

Preheat oven to 400°F (200°C). Shake marinade from chicken, lightly blotting excess moisture with a paper towel. Place in oiled cast iron pan and bake for 40 minutes until skin is just starting to brown. Remove from pan—it is okay if the chicken is not totally done—you will be finishing it on top of the croutons once they are crisp.

Toss bread cubes in pan with chicken juice and fat, add a generous sprinkle of salt, the caper berries, and the remaining chopped herbs. If croutons seem dry add 1 tablespoon of olive oil to coat. Bake until croutons are crisp around edges, about 20 minutes. Toss halfway through so they crisp evenly.

Place chicken on top of bread and heat for another 15–20 minutes until skin is crisp and chicken is cooked through.

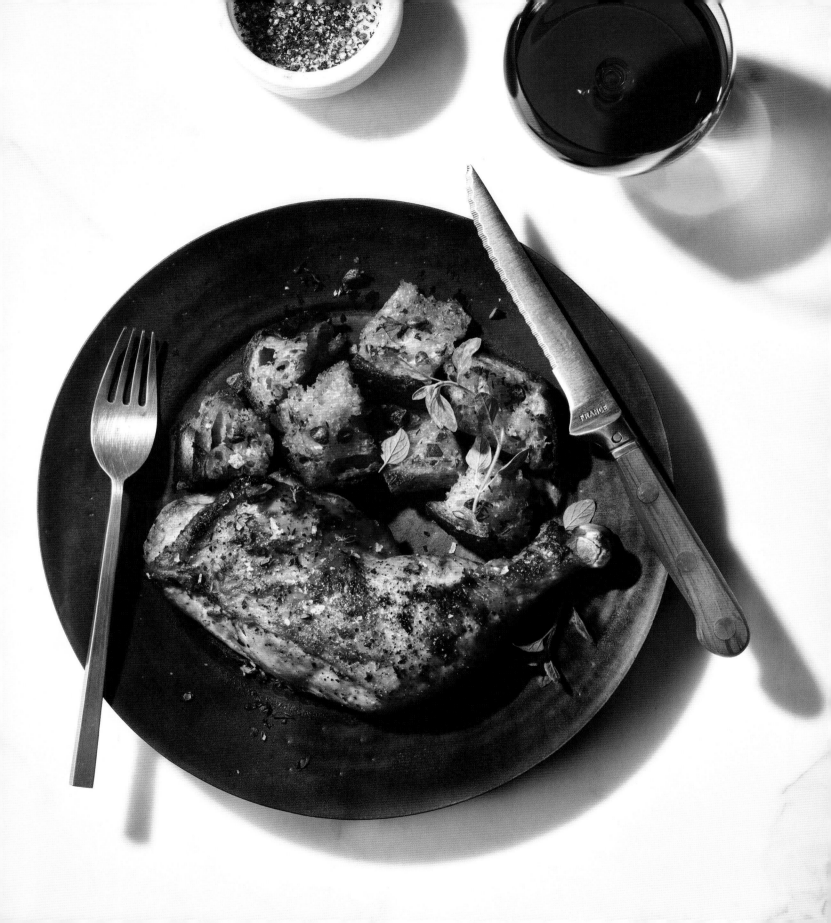

# pulled pork

**MAKES 1 ½ QUARTS** | LF | GF

An excellent go-to recipe when cooking for a big group—the trick to it is to cook on the stovetop after the oven so that the liquid can reduce and absorb back into the shredded meat. This can be made up to two days ahead of time and can also be cooked overnight in a slow cooker then finished up on the stove. Rule of thumb is ½ – ¾ pound of meat per person and this recipe can easily be scaled up if you have a bigger party. Serve with warm tortillas, lime wedges, and thinly sliced radishes. Also, it makes great sandwiches.

## INGREDIENTS

3 pounds pork shoulder, preferably pasture raised

2 teaspoons ground coriander

2 teaspoons smoked paprika

2 tablespoons oregano

2 teaspoons garlic powder

2 teaspoons salt

½ teaspoon cayenne

½ teaspoon cinnamon

1 tablespoon olive oil

Juice of 1 orange

2 tablespoons rice vinegar

Ground black pepper

## PREPARATION

One hour before cooking, combine spices and salt and rub on all sides of the pork.

Preheat oven to 325°F (180°C). In a Dutch oven, heat the oil and sear the pork on all sides over medium-high heat, cooking 5–8 minutes to create a light crust before turning. After searing each side, add orange juice and rice vinegar, scrape brown bits from the bottom then cover pot and transfer to the oven.

Cook 2½ hours, flipping pork over in pan and rotating pan halfway through cooking. Remove from oven and break meat into large chunks. Place pan, uncovered, on stovetop over medium heat breaking pieces into smaller chunks as they simmer. Continue cooking for about 30 minutes while periodically breaking into smaller and smaller pieces with two forks until juice has just absorbed into meat so the meat is tender and shredded.

Season with salt, vinegar, and cayenne and black pepper to taste.

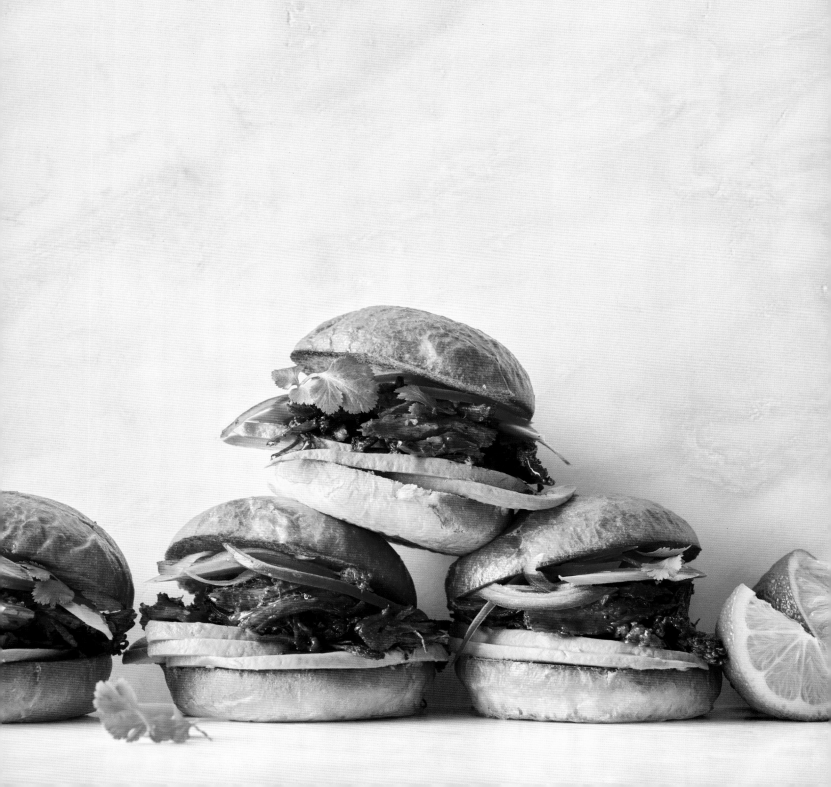

# white wine halibut *with* vegetables

**SERVES 6–7** | LF | GF

My daughter and I came up with this recipe recently. There was beautiful halibut at our local fish market, so armed with the fresh fish and a bag of spinach, we went home to see what we could concoct. We already had a box of mushrooms and cherry tomatoes in the refrigerator, and I always keep green onions and white wine on hand, so we put our heads together and came up with this. It was a great night, mom and daughter cooking together and we created one of my new favorite dishes—low fat, heart healthy, full of vitamins, minerals, and antioxidants. And delicious!

## INGREDIENTS

1 pound mushrooms (I use a mix of shiitake and crimini), quartered

Olive oil

1 pint cherry tomatoes, halved

Small handful chopped capers or caper berries

5 green onions, thinly sliced

¾ cups inexpensive dry white wine (I use a Sauvignon Blanc)

1 bunch parsley chopped

2 teaspoons Dijon mustard

½ pounds of fresh halibut, skin removed (you can substitute any firm fish for this recipe)

2 bags triple washed spinach

Sea salt and ground black pepper, to taste

## PREPARATION

In extra large sauté pan over medium heat, cook mushrooms in a generous amount of olive oil with a few pinches of salt until the edges start to crisp, about 15 minutes. Turn up heat, add cherry tomatoes, capers, half the sliced green onions, another pinch of salt then cook until cherry tomatoes start to have a little color, about 3 minutes. Add white wine, parsley and mustard, and scrape brown bits off bottom of pan.

Season the fish with sea salt and pepper on both sides, move mushroom mixture to side of pan, add the fish and cover. Lower heat to medium and cook for 3 to 4 minutes on each side. Spoon mushroom mixture over top of fish after you flip to second side, adding more wine if needed.

In a separate pan, sauté remaining green onions and spinach over medium heat for two minutes. When the spinach is wilted but not totally cooked add it to the pan with the fish.

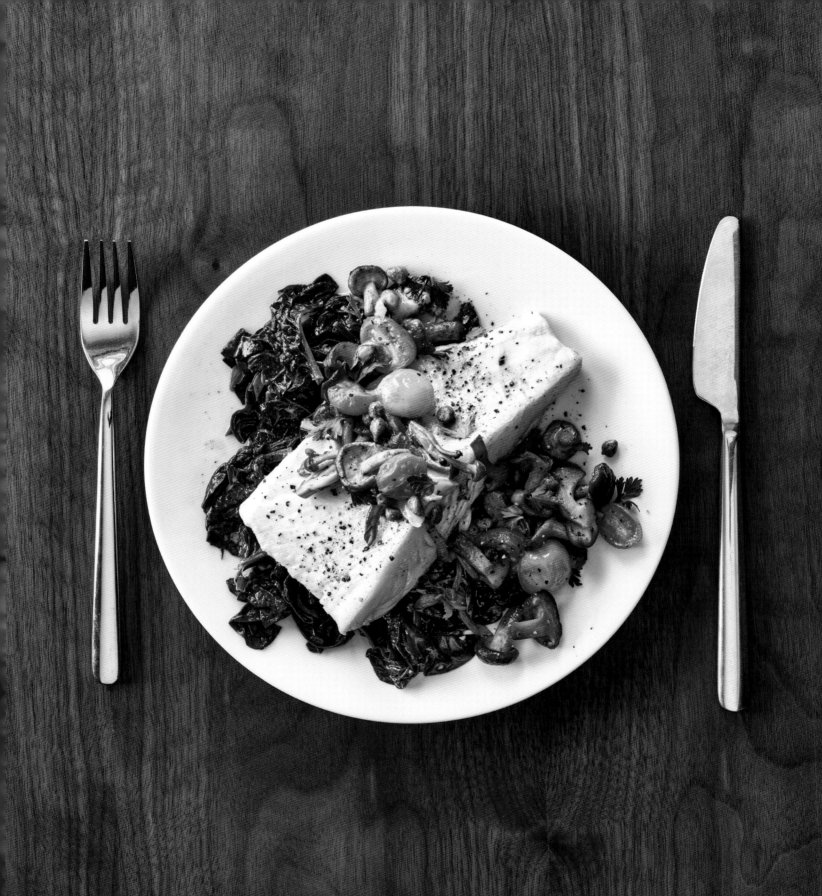

# mussels three ways

**SERVES 6 AS A STARTER** | LF | GF

Mussels are an elegant start to a meal and are super easy to prepare. They can live out of water for two to three days in the refrigerator in a bowl or baking dish with a bag full of ice covered with a paper towel.

When you are ready to cook, place mussels in a colander under running water and tap each shell to make sure it closes. Discard all mussels that do not close after tapping or that have cracked shells. If they were not debearded by the fishmonger, you can do so by pulling the small clump that rests on the edge of the shell by grabbing firmly and pulling downward.

When cooking it is very important to season these well. Since these recipes call for so many mussels, make sure to season accordingly with more salt and pepper than you may think so the broth is flavorful. Serve with grilled bread or Crispy Fingerling Potatoes (p. 63).

# mussels *with* tomato, shallots & white wine

## INGREDIENTS

2 tablespoons olive oil

3 shallots, diced

Salt and ground black pepper, to taste

5 tomatoes, diced

Pinch chili flakes

Pinch saffron

2 cups dry white wine

2 cups water or fish stock

72 mussels, scrubbed and debearded (about 2½ pounds)

1 tablespoon parsley, minced for garnish

## PREPARATION

In a large pot over medium heat, heat olive oil and sauté shallots for about 3 minutes with a pinch of salt and pepper. Add tomatoes and chili flakes and cook for 3 minutes more. Add saffron, wine, water (or stock), mussels, and a couple generous pinches of salt and pepper. Lower heat and cover. Cook for about 3 minutes or until mussels open. Discard any mussels that do not open. Season to taste.

## TO SERVE:

Place mussels in individual bowls (12 per bowl). Ladle broth on top and garnish with parsley.

# coconut & lemongrass mussels

## INGREDIENTS

4 shallots (or two red onions), diced

3 tablespoons ginger, minced

6 stalks lemongrass, thinly sliced

3 tablespoons olive oil

8 cloves garlic, minced

Juice of 3 limes

2 cans (15 ounces each) coconut milk

72 mussels, scrubbed and debearded (about 2½ pounds)

½ cup water

Salt and ground black pepper, to taste

Scallions, thinly sliced for garnish

## PREPARATION

In large pot over medium heat, sauté shallots, ginger, and lemongrass in olive oil with a generous pinch of salt and pepper for about 5 minutes. Add garlic and cook for a minute more. Add lime and coconut milk until hot. Add mussels then lower heat and cover. Cook for about 3 minutes or until mussels open. Discard any mussels that do not open. Season with generous pinches of salt and pepper to taste.

## TO SERVE:

Arrange mussels in individual bowls (12 per person). Ladle broth on top and garnish with scallions.

# fennel & garlic butter mussels

## INGREDIENTS

2 tablespoons olive oil

2 fennel bulbs, diced

Salt and ground black pepper, to taste

4 garlic cloves, thinly sliced

3 cups dry white wine

3 cups water

72 mussels, scrubbed and debearded (about 2½ pounds)

3 tablespoons butter

2 tablespoons dried or fresh tarragon, minced

2 tablespoons fennel fronds, minced for garnish

## PREPARATION

In large pot over medium heat, heat olive oil and sauté fennel with a generous pinch of salt and pepper for about 6–8 minutes until soft. Add garlic for last 3 minutes of cooking. Add wine, water, salt and pepper, and let come to a boil. Add mussels then lower heat and cover. Cook for about 3 minutes until mussels open. Discard any mussels that do not open. Stir in butter and tarragon and season to taste.

## TO SERVE:

Arrange mussels in individual bowls (12 per person). Ladle broth on top and garnish with fennel fronds.

# Henry's baked cinnamon twists *with* chocolate sauce

**MAKES APPROXIMATELY 18 TWISTS** | LF | V

This sweet treat is made with leftover Pizza Dough (p. 105) and has been a long-time family favorite.

### INGREDIENTS

½ batch of Pizza Dough (p. 105)

2 tablespoons coconut oil or butter, melted

3 tablespoons sugar

1 tablespoon cinnamon

Chocolate Sauce (p. 92)

### PREPARATION

Preheat oven to 350°F (180°C). Roll dough into a large rectangle about ¼" thick. Brush with coconut oil and sprinkle with 2 tablespoons of the cinnamon and sugar mixture. Cut into ½" strips. Fold each strip in half and twist. Lay finished strips on large parchment-lined sheet pan about 2" apart. Brush twists with coconut oil and dust with remaining cinnamon and sugar. Bake for 12 minutes until lightly golden brown.

While twists are baking, warm chocolate sauce on stove. Serve finished twists with small bowls of chocolate sauce for dipping.

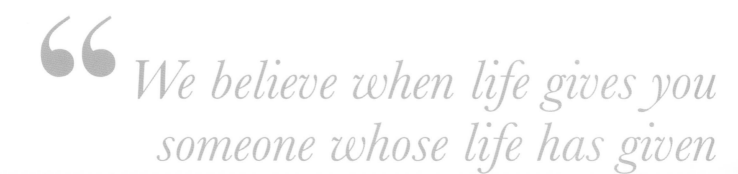

*We believe when life gives you someone whose life has given*

# pomegranate granita

**MAKES 6 CUPS** | LF | V | GF

The simplicity of this granita is unmatched. The juice of the pomegranate is sweet and tangy, and full of nutrients. As a frozen treat, it's perfect after a rich autumn meal.

### INGREDIENTS

5 cups pomegranate juice

1 cup water

3 tablespoons maple syrup (to taste)

### PREPARATION

Combine all ingredients in a 9 × 13" baking dish. Place in the freezer for 3 hours. Every 30 minutes, use a fork to break up and scrape clumps of ice that begin to form.

# vegan peanut butter ice cream

**MAKES 1 QUART** | LF | V | GF
Adapted from *Vegan Ice Cream by Jeff Rogers*

You won't feel guilty about enjoying this egg-free and dairy-free frozen delight. With easily available ingredients and very little preparation, you can have a decadent dessert any night of the week.

### INGREDIENTS

1 cup raw cashews

1 cup creamy peanut butter

½ cup maple syrup (or to taste)

2 teaspoons vanilla extract

⅛ teaspoon almond extract

2 cups water

### PREPARATION

Blend all ingredients in blender for 2 minutes until completely smooth. Freeze or refrigerate mixture for an hour until well chilled. Pour mix into ice cream maker and freeze according to your ice cream maker's instructions. Can be served immediately or frozen in an airtight container until ready to serve.

*lemons, you should try to find them vodka and make limoncellos.* "

# chocolate coconut cashew mousse

**MAKES 1 ½ CUPS** | LF | V | GF

Here's a dressed up version of the simple Cashew Cream for when you want something a little more decadent.

---

### INGREDIENTS

1½ cup cashews, soaked 1 hour in water and drained

⅓ cup water + more if needed to make creamy

1 teaspoon vanilla extract

1 teaspoon coconut oil

3 tablespoons maple syrup

3 tablespoons unsweetened cocoa powder

¼ teaspoon salt

### TOPPINGS:

1 pint mixed berries

Dark chocolate, shaved

Mint, for garnish

### PREPARATION

Combine all ingredients in a high powered blender or food processor and blend until smooth and creamy. Add more water as needed. Serve topped with berries, shaved chocolate, and mint leaf garnish.

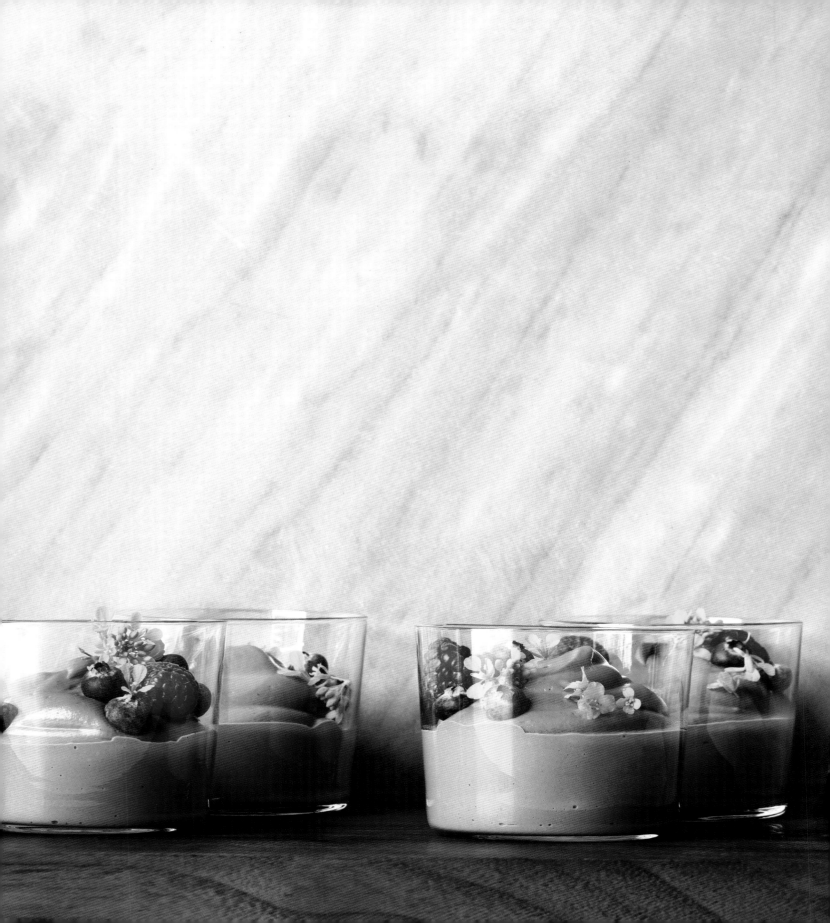

# pistachio baklava rolls

**MAKES 24 ROLLS** | LF | V

Adapted from *My Moroccan Food*

Crispy and sweet, these make a great afternoon tea treat or after dinner treat with coffee or tea. They sound complicated but actually come together quickly so they can be made last minute. Phyllo typically comes in packages of 20 sheets and can be thawed and refrozen. You can divide the thawed sheets into smaller packages of 4 sheets each before refreezing. That way, you won't have to keep defrosting and refreezing the whole package when you need only a few sheets at a time. Covering with a wet paper towel keeps the sheets from getting crumbly. I overlap a couple paper towels to make sure the edges stay covered. You can brush the oil on or use your hands, gently smoothing the oil from edge to edge.

## INGREDIENTS

**FILLING:**

1¾ cups pistachios or mix of pecans, almonds, walnuts and/or pistachios

Pinch each of cardamom, cinnamon, and coriander

3 tablespoons caster sugar

½ teaspoon salt

3 tablespoons orange blossom water or vanilla extract

1 tablespoon coconut oil

**SYRUP:**

½ cup maple syrup

Pinch each of cardamom, cinnamon, and coriander

½ teaspoon orange blossom water or vanilla extract

3 drops sesame oil

Generous pinches of salt

½ cup walnut oil or olive oil

2 tablespoons nuts, finely chopped, for garnish

**ROLLS:**

8 sheets phyllo, package defrosted in refrigerator overnight

## PREPARATION

Preheat oven to 350°F (180°C). Blend all ingredients for filling in a food processor until it becomes a cohesive, somewhat smooth paste. (This can be made a few days in advance and kept in the refrigerator.) Roll paste into four tubes that are as long as the short side of the phyllo dough.

Unwrap phyllo dough and cover with a damp paper towel. Brush one sheet of dough with oil and place another sheet on top. Brush sheet with oil. Lay tube of paste along short edge of dough and roll into long cylindrical shape. Brush outside with oil, set aside, and repeat with remaining phyllo and pistachio paste.

Line up the four pastry tubes and cut into sixths (you will end up with 24 little rolls). Place rolls on parchment-lined baking sheet and bake for 20 minutes or until tops and bottoms are golden. The bottoms brown more quickly than the tops so check to make sure bottoms aren't burning.

While pastry is baking combine all syrup ingredients and whisk.

When rolls are golden and crispy, remove from oven and pour syrup over top, turning them over every couple minutes until syrup has absorbed into pastry. Top with minced nuts and serve.

# whoopie pies *with* coconut cream

**MAKES 6 (3 ½") COOKIE SANDWICHES** | LF | V
Adapted from *Woman's Day*

Whoopie pies are a New England favorite. This unconventional version substitutes coconut whipped cream for the traditional marshmallow fluff or buttercream.

## INGREDIENTS

**COOKIES:**

1 cup sugar

½ cup coconut oil

1½ teaspoons baking soda

½ teaspoon baking powder

½ teaspoon salt

½ cup cocoa powder

1 egg

1 teaspoon vanilla extract

1 cup almond milk

2 cups all-purpose flour

**FILLING:**

4 cans (5.4 ounces each) coconut cream, refrigerated overnight

1 teaspoon powdered sugar

1 teaspoon vanilla extract

## PREPARATION

Preheat oven 375°F (190°C). In a large bowl with an electric or stand mixer, cream sugar, coconut oil, baking soda, baking powder, and salt until well combined and slightly fluffy. About 2 minutes. Add cocoa, egg, and vanilla extract then whip until smooth. On low speed, alternately mix in flour and milk until you have a thick batter. The consistency will be a little softer than a typical cookie dough and a little thicker than a cake batter.

Cover a large sheet pan or two small sheet pans with parchment and drop scant ¼ cup scoops 3" apart. Make sure you leave plenty of room between them, as they spread. Bake for 15 minutes until slightly firm to the touch. Let cool completely before filling.

While cookies are baking, prepare filling by scooping the solid coconut cream into a medium-sized bowl or bowl of a stand mixer. Reserve 1 teaspoon of the coconut liquid. Add vanilla extract and powdered sugar to solid coconut cream and beat on high until fluffy. If cream is lumpy add reserved liquid ¼ teaspoon at a time. Too much liquid and your coconut whipped cream will be too runny. When cookies are cooled, divide coconut cream between 6 halves. Spread into an even layer and top with second cookie. Refrigerate for 15 minutes before serving so whipped cream can set.

These can be refrigerated in an airtight container for 3 days.

# lemon, ginger & thyme vodka

**SERVES 8** | LF | V | GF

Have this brisk and flavorful syrup at-the-ready for entertaining. Lemon, thyme, and ginger —three distinct flavors that mix surprisingly well together. Serve chilled or as a hot toddy.

---

### INGREDIENTS

Lemon juice

Vodka

Ice cubes

### HONEY, GINGER, AND THYME SYRUP:

½ cup honey

½ cup water

3" piece ginger, sliced thin

10 thyme sprigs

### PREPARATION

To make syrup place honey, water, ginger, and thyme in a small saucepan. Bring to a boil, lower heat and simmer over low heat for about 30 minutes. Let cool for 20–25 minutes and strain. Add enough water to replace water that evaporated during simmering to bring syrup to 1 cup.

### FOR A CHILLED DRINK:

In a cocktail glass, fill with ice, add 1½ ounces vodka, 1 ounce syrup, and 1 ounce lemon juice then stir.

If making a large batch of drinks, you can mix 1 cup syrup, 1 cup lemon juice, and 1½ cups vodka.

### FOR A HOT TODDY-STYLE DRINK:

Warm syrup. In a mug, add 2 ounces vodka, 1½ ounces syrup, 1½ ounces lemon juice, and hot water to taste.

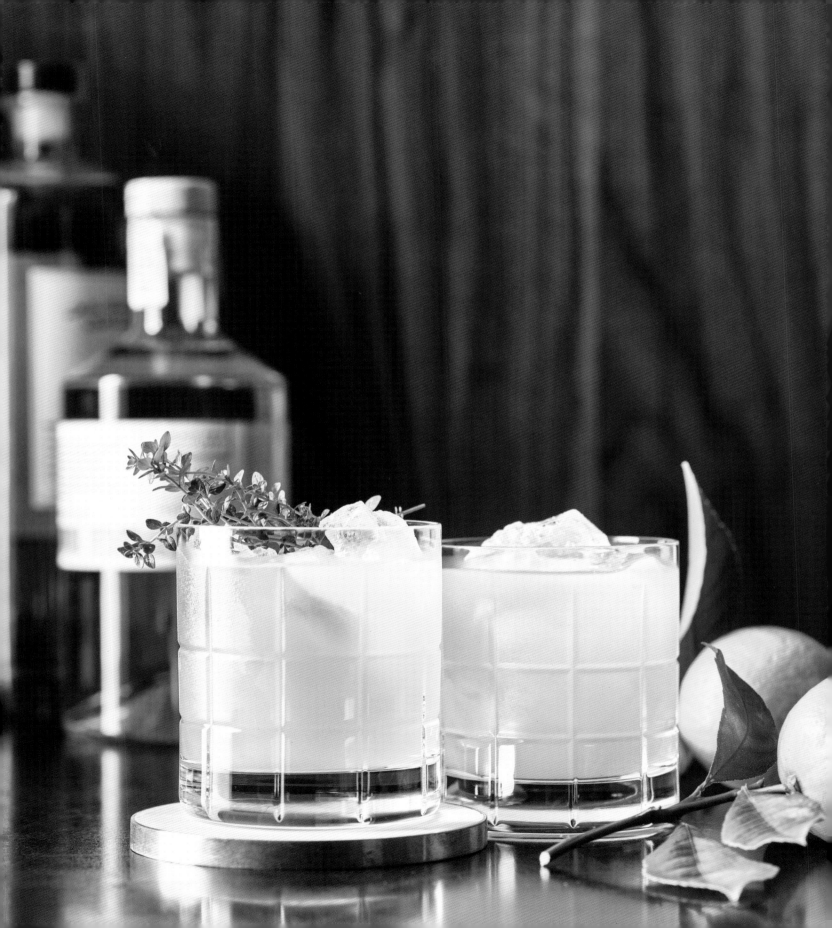

# sage tea

**MAKES 1 CUP** | LF | V | GF

This is one of my favorite teas to drink in the fall, so soothing when the weather gets chilly. I usually keep fresh sage in the refrigerator for all of my fall cooking.

---

**INGREDIENTS**

Sage leaves

**PREPARATION**

Just throw a few leaves in a mug and cover with boiling water. Steep for 5 minutes.

> *Fresh sage leaves can be used to soothe insect bites and, it's claimed, can whiten teeth. We like them in a mug of tea next to a fire.*

# spiked spicy hot cocoa

**MAKES 1 DRINK** | LF | V | GF

Here's something cozy for snuggling up in front of the fireplace.

## INGREDIENTS

1½ cups lactose-free milk (use your favorite)

2 tablespoons Chocolate Sauce (p. 92)

1–2 ounces Chai-Infused Vodka (below)

## PREPARATION

Heat milk in saucepan with chocolate syrup until hot. Pour into mug and stir in vodka. Top with cinnamon.

You can also make a peppermint hot cocoa by substituting plain vodka and adding a drop of peppermint oil or ½ teaspoon of peppermint extract.

# chai-infused vodka

**MAKES 2 CUPS** | LF | V | GF

The sweet, aromatic flavors of cardamom and cinnamon are balanced with the bite of the ginger and the heat of the peppercorns. The deep and complex flavor profile is unique and perfect for autumn evenings.

## INGREDIENTS

2 cups vodka

1 cinnamon stick

4 green cardamom pods

1" piece of ginger, peeled

5 peppercorns

## PREPARATION

Pour vodka over spices in a pint jar with a tight-fitting lid. Steep for 5 days shaking daily. Strain and store in clean jar.

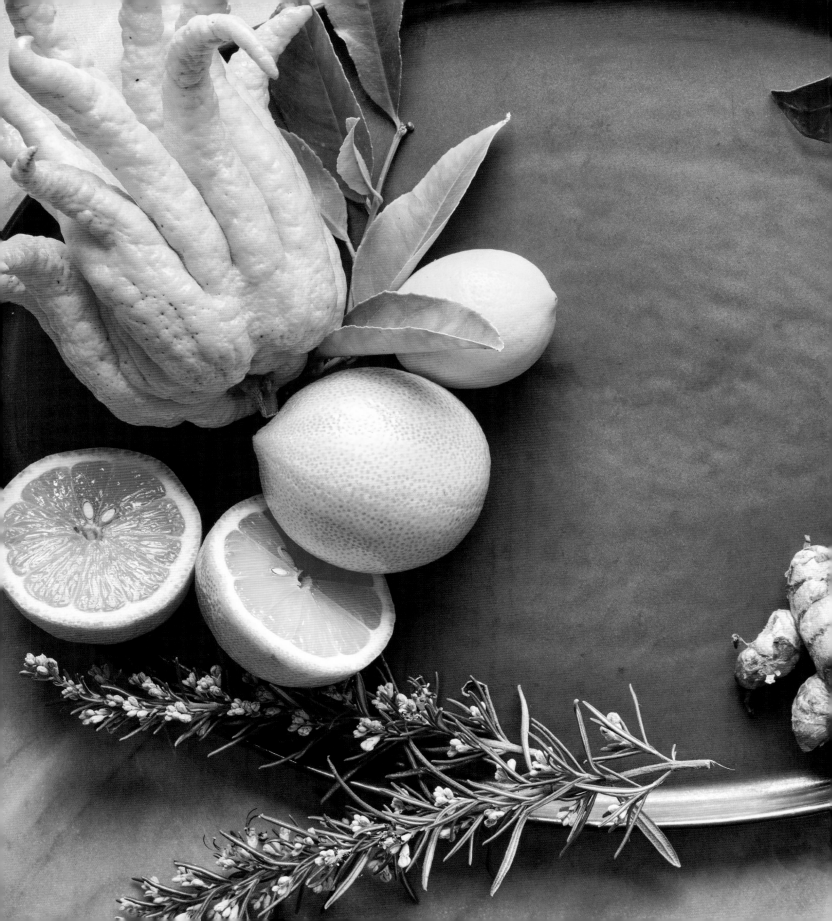

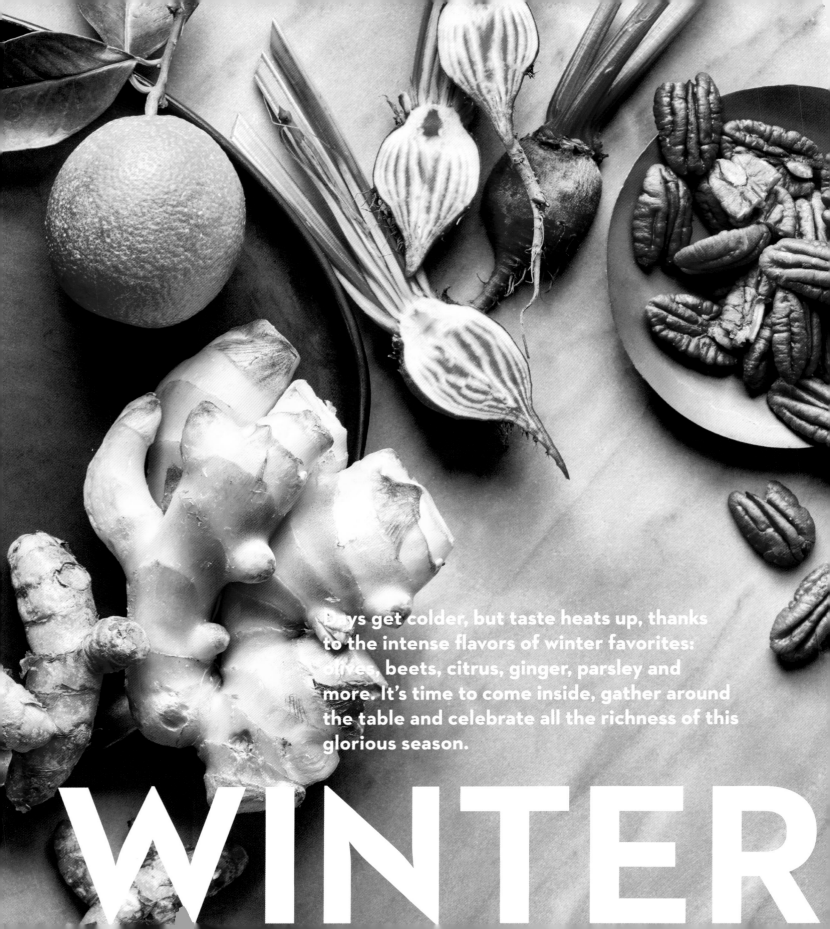

Days get colder, but taste heats up, thanks to the intense flavors of winter favorites: olives, beets, citrus, ginger, parsley and more. It's time to come inside, gather around the table and celebrate all the richness of this glorious season.

# WINTER

It's time to celebrate! Parties, gatherings, family get-togethers, big events—they're all on the calendar. Balancing the fun and your microbiome is easy when you find moments of quiet in the chaos to calm your digestive system. Enjoy every satisfying bite of winter's SIBO-friendly dishes that support you through the happiest time of the year.

# winter mushroom & gruyère frittata

**MAKES 1 (12") FRITTATA** | LF | V | GF

Enjoy this earthy and comforting dish on chilly days.

## INGREDIENTS

1 red onion, diced

½ pound crimini mushrooms
(or a mix of whatever mushrooms
you like) thinly sliced

1 cup grated Gruyère cheese, grated

10 sage leaves, minced

1 tablespoon thyme, minced

1 tablespoon ghee

12 eggs + 1 can (5.4 ounces) coconut
cream + 1¼ teaspoon of salt blended
in blender or with hand blender
until frothy

## PREPARATION

Preheat oven to 400°F (200°C). Sauté red onion, herbs, mushrooms, and a few pinches of salt over medium-high heat with ghee until mushrooms are brown around edges. Top with half of the cheese.

While pan is over low heat, pour in half of the egg mixture, top with remaining cheese, and pour in remaining egg mixture. Cook on stovetop until edges of frittata start to set.

Bake for 15 minutes until middle of frittata is almost completely set. It will continue to firm up over next 10 minutes.

# C'EST CHEESE

*Lactose is a SIBO no-no, but fortunately you can still enjoy cheese. The key is choosing low-lactose or lactose-free cheeses, of which there are several wonderful varieties of hard-aged cheeses to choose from. While the choices are fewer, cheese is still an excellent ingredient for those with SIBO. Cheese is high in bone-building calcium, a nutrient often lacking in American diets. Cheese is also a fantastic source of protein (and easy to pack). It also contains a plethora of important vitamin and minerals, like Vitamin B12, riboflavin, and zinc. Definitely take a pass on the brie, and follow these tips to enjoying the cheese course without regret:*

---

- Stick to hard-aged cheeses such as Parmesan, Pecorino, hard Cheddar, and other aged cheeses like Manchego. Gruyère is the SIBO-standout, as it's 100% lactose-free.

- Be mindful of portion-size, even low-lactose cheese can have a cumulative effect if eaten in large quantities; one serving per meal is best.

- For easiest digestion, aim to eat just one type of cheese at any mealtime. Two can be tolerated if in smaller portions.

# almond & sesame grain-free granola

**MAKES 3 CUPS** | LF | V | GF

Crunchy and grain-free, this is a satisfying breakfast staple to keep in your pantry.

## INGREDIENTS

2 tablespoons coconut oil

1 cup raw sliced almonds

½ cup raw sunflower seeds

½ cup pumpkin seeds

¼ cup sesame seeds

⅓ cup unsweetened shredded coconut

3 tablespoons maple syrup

Zest of ½ lemon

Pinch each nutmeg, cardamom, and cinnamon

Salt to taste

## PREPARATION

Heat coconut oil in large sauté pan over medium-high heat. Add almonds and toast while stirring for 3 minutes, add sunflower seeds and toast for another couple minutes. Then add sesame seeds and coconut and toast until everything is starting to brown. Add maple syrup, lemon zest, spices, and two generous pinches of salt. Cook until maple syrup makes a sticky coating, about 1 minute more.

Spread cooked granola onto a sheet pan, sprinkle with crunchy salt and let cool. When completely cooled store in an airtight container.

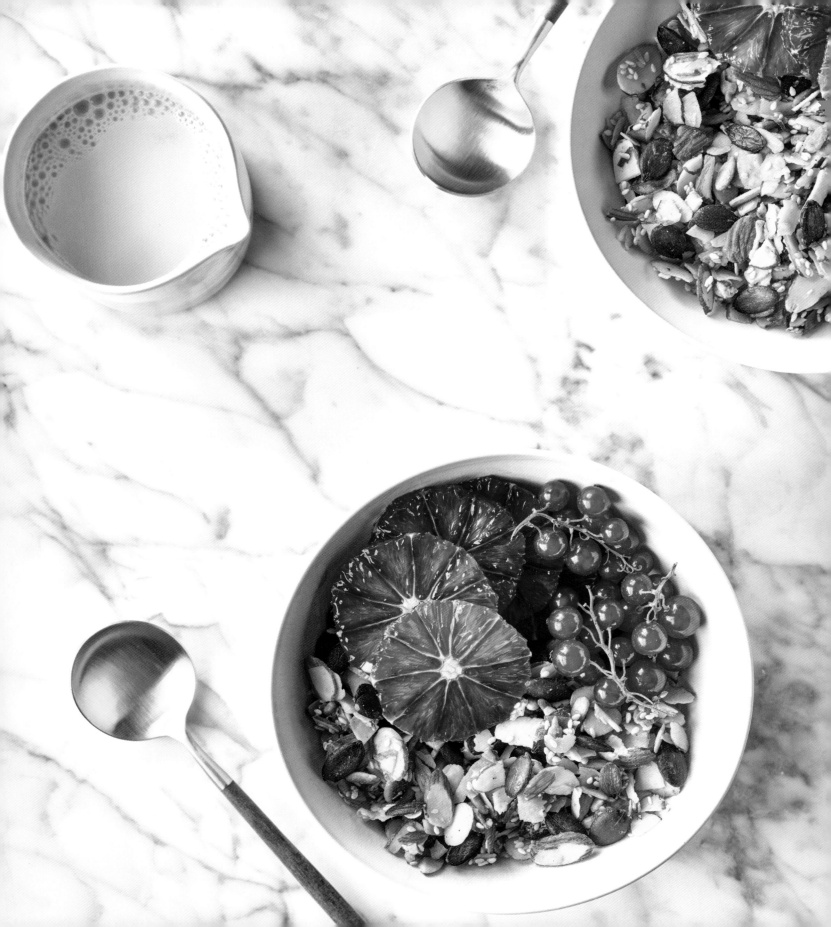

# easy marinated olives

**SERVES 4** | LF | V | GF

Here's something quick and pretty to throw together for unexpected guests or an added nibble for a cocktail party.

### INGREDIENTS

½ jar pitted green olives, drained

½ jar pitted Kalamata olives, drained

Peel of 1 lemon and/or orange using a vegetable peeler

Juice of ½ lemon and/or orange

1 bay leaf

1 teaspoon toasted ground fennel seed

Pinch red pepper flakes

Enough olive oil to cover olives

### PREPARATION

Add everything to a small saucepan and heat for 10 minutes over low heat. Serve warm with crusty bread to dip in oil.

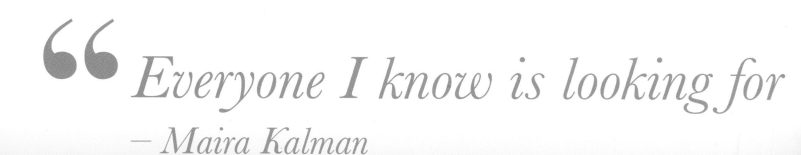

" *Everyone I know is looking for*

— *Maira Kalman*

# bar nuts

**SERVES 4** | LF | V | GF

This is one of those recipes that is barely a recipe at all. It's more of a quick something to take to a party or to have around as a snack, and it's more interesting than a handful of raw nuts. Add more sugar if you want a sweeter mix, cayenne pepper if you want it spicy. It can be made with any combination of nuts you may have in your pantry and whatever herbs and spices sound interesting. I like to add enough oil that they leave my fingers oily after I eat them.

---

### INGREDIENTS

Large handful each of raw almonds, pepitas, and pecans (or whatever combination of nuts/seeds you have)

Generous dusting of smoked paprika, sugar, and salt

Enough olive oil to generously coat nuts

Dried ground rosemary

### PREPARATION

Heat oven to 300°F (150°C) and mix everything together on a parchment-lined sheet pan. Roast slowly in oven for 20 minutes.

*solace, hope and a tasty snack.* "

# kalamata olive basil tapenade

**MAKES 1 ½ CUPS** | LF | V | GF

Here's a quick and flavorful tapenade. It's great on crostini and can be added to hot pasta for an easy weeknight supper.

### INGREDIENTS

½ cup pitted Kalamata olives

½ cup pitted green olives

1 cup loosely packed basil

¼ cup loosely packed parsley leaves

Large pinch sea salt

Large pinch ground black pepper

Zest of one lemon

2 teaspoons lemon juice

1 teaspoon white wine vinegar

3 tablespoons garlic-infused olive oil

### PREPARATION

Combine all ingredients in the bowl of a food processor. Pulse until all herbs and olives are finely chopped, but not completely puréed, scraping down the sides of the bowl a few times. Adjust seasoning to taste.

# anchovy parsley tapenade

**MAKES ⅓ CUP** | LF | V | GF

This tapenade makes a terrific spread for crackers or bread—if you have any leftover, add it to a sandwich. Don't let the anchovies deter you from trying this recipe, they are not overpowering and they blend beautifully with the other ingredients. The roasted almonds add a toothsome texture to this delectable spread.

### INGREDIENTS

¼ cup almonds, toasted

½ cup tightly packed parsley leaves

5 anchovy fillets

3 tablespoons olive oil

1 ½ teaspoons white wine vinegar

1 teaspoon lemon juice

Zest of 1 lemon

⅛ teaspoon ground black pepper

Salt to taste (add at the end because anchovies are salty)

### PREPARATION

Combine all ingredients (except salt) in the bowl of a food processor. Pulse until almonds and herbs are finely chopped, but not completely puréed, scraping down the sides of the bowl a few times. Adjust seasoning to taste.

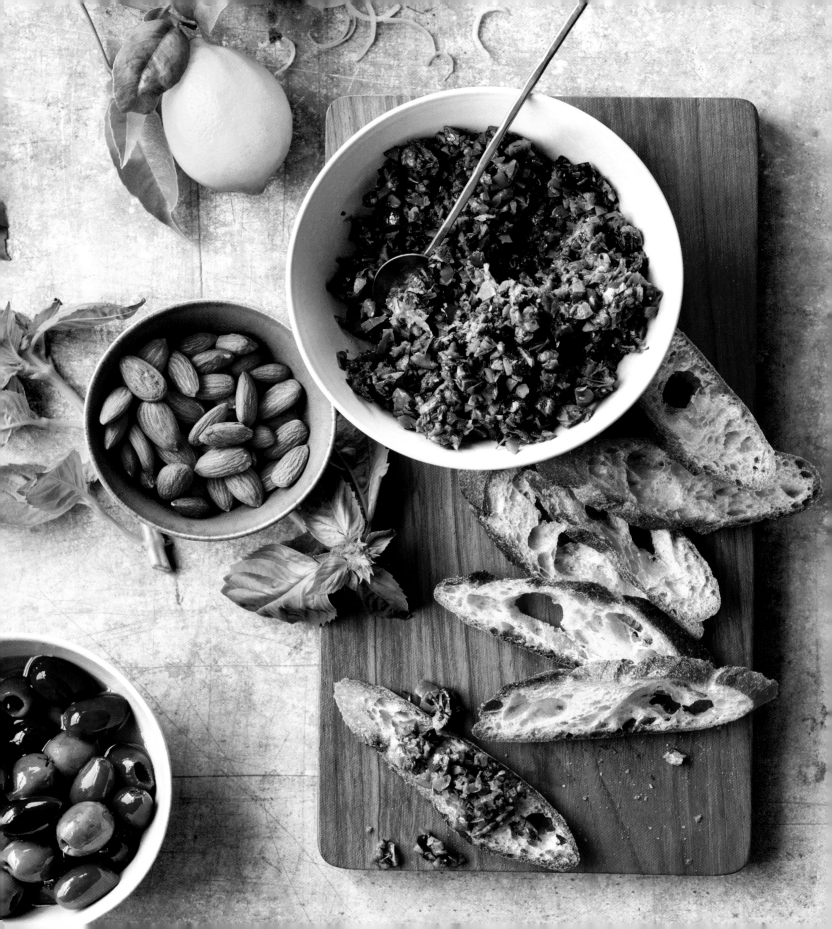

# cashew spinach spanakopita

**MAKES 12–16 SMALL TRIANGLES** | V

Traditional spanakopita uses feta cheese, but for this recipe we are enlisting cashews instead. The soaked and blended cashews, with help from lemon juice and salt, are a dairy-free stand-in for cheese. The layers of flaky pastry and spinach filling are simply scrumptious.

## INGREDIENTS

1 box phyllo dough

1 cup cashews, soaked

1 bunch cilantro, roughly chopped and wilted with spinach

¾ pound spinach, wilted with water pressed out

1 bunch scallions, roughly chopped

¾ cup Kalamata olives, roughly chopped

Juice and zest of 1 lemon

½ cup walnut oil, or olive oil or melted ghee

½ cup Parmesan cheese, grated (optional)

3 onions diced then caramelized until reduced to 1 cup

2 pinches each: coriander, nutmeg, and black pepper added to onions while caramelizing

Salt to taste

## PREPARATION

The night before you make the spanakopita, leave phyllo dough package in refrigerator to defrost overnight. Bring it to room temperature for 30 minutes before use.

In a food processor, pulse cashews until roughly chopped. Add cilantro, spinach, scallions, olives, lemon juice and zest, and pulse until combined. It should still have texture so don't purée. Scrape into a bowl, stir in onions and season to taste.

Lay one sheet of phyllo out on a board, brush with oil or melted ghee. Place another sheet on top and brush with oil or ghee. Cut into six strips width-wise. Place a heaping tablespoon of filling on bottom corner of each strip and fold into triangle shaped packages. Brush tops with oil.

Place on baking rack on baking sheet and bake for 35–40 minutes rotating after 15 minutes until golden brown and crispy.

# focaccia

**MAKES 1 (13 × 9") FOCACCIA** | V

Focaccia is one of my favorite breads. It's great for panini, alongside steamed mussels, or with a few spoonfuls of pesto for dipping as an appetizer. Don't skimp on the olive oil—this is what gives it flavor and a crispy bottom.

### INGREDIENTS

Pizza Dough (p. 105)

½ cup olive oil, divided in half

2 tablespoons rosemary, chopped

Crunchy salt

### PREPARATION

Make 1 batch of Pizza Dough (p. 105), adding rosemary to flour before mixing. Follow dough recipe, adding a few more minutes of kneading to build gluten, so about 5 minutes. Instead of dividing into separate balls, place entire ball of dough in a large oiled mixing bowl. Like the pizza dough, this dough can be made up to three days ahead of time and improves each day. If you are using the dough right away, cover bowl with damp towel and let dough rise in warm place until doubled in size, about 1 hour.

If you are making dough ahead of time, cover bowl tightly with plastic wrap and let dough rise slowly in the refrigerator, push it down each day to make sure it doesn't escape the container. On the day you are using the dough, do not push down, you want it to have a full rise when you use it.

When you are ready to make your bread, preheat oven to 400°F (200°C) and liberally oil a sheet pan with ¼ cup olive oil. Tip dough onto sheet pan and use your hands to spread dough to edges of pan. If dough is pulling back towards the center let dough rest for 20 minutes and spread again. When dough is spread to edges of pan, cover with towel, parchment, or plastic wrap and let rise until doubled in size, or about 1 hour.

Use your fingers to make dimples over the entire surface of risen dough and pour remaining olive oil over top of dough, filling each indentation and adding additional oil if there are any empty indentations.

Bake bread on middle rack of oven for 30–45 minutes until top is nice and golden, rotating pan halfway through. Top finished bread with crunchy salt.

# leftover risotto arancini

**MAKES 12 (2") BALLS** | GF

I like to make extra Weeknight Risotto (p. 191) just so I can have leftovers to make arancini. They are good on their own or dipped in marinara, salsa verde, or pesto. You can make risotto just to make arancini but it needs to be refrigerated until cold before rolling into balls.

## INGREDIENTS

4 cups leftover Weeknight Risotto (p. 191)

2 cups Parmesan cheese, grated

4 eggs, beaten

2 cups flour, seasoned with salt and pepper

2 cups bread crumbs or almond meal (for gluten-free)

½ pound Gruyère cheese, cut into ½" cubes

Neutral high heat oil like grapeseed or sunflower

## PREPARATION

Fold Parmesan into cold risotto. On separate plates, lay out your flour, bread crumbs, and eggs. Have two sheet pans ready, one for coated rice balls and one lined with paper towels for after frying. Roll rice ball into 2" balls. To fill them, press a your finger into the center, place a cube of cheese and carefully cover hole. Roll rice ball in eggs then flour, then again in eggs and into the bread crumbs, then set onto sheet pan.

Once all of the balls are coated, heat 1" of oil in a large heavy-bottomed skillet. The oil is ready when a bread crumb sizzles around the edges. Fill pan with coated rice balls making sure they are not too crowded, cook on each side making sure they are evenly golden brown. Turn down heat if they are browning too quickly or unevenly. They should cook for about 10–15 minutes total. When finished, place on sheet pan lined with paper towel and sprinkle with crunchy salt.

# crab cakes *with* simple cornichon remoulade

**MAKES 12 (3") CAKES** | LF | GF

Almond meal and a few shrimp ground into a sticky paste hold these crab cakes together without overpowering the crab's natural sweetness. Use the highest quality crab you can and be sure to pick out any shell.

## INGREDIENTS

### CRAB CAKES:

¼ pound shrimp, shells removed (about 5–6 large shrimp)

1 egg

1 tablespoon mayonnaise

1 tablespoon Dijon mustard

2 stalks celery, finely diced

2 tablespoons parsley, minced

1 heaping teaspoon Old Bay Seasoning

1 pound crab meat

⅔ cup almond meal

Sunflower oil, or grapeseed oil or ghee for frying

### REMOULADE:

10 cornichons, finely minced

4 tablespoons mayonnaise

½ teaspoon Old Bay Seasoning

### TO SERVE:

2 tablespoons parsley or chives, minced

## PREPARATION

In the bowl of a food processor or with a knife, chop shrimp finely until it becomes a sticky paste.

In a large bowl, mix shrimp paste with egg, mayonnaise, Dijon mustard, celery, parsley, and Old Bay Seasoning. Fold in crab. Sprinkle almond meal on top and gently mix.

Heat 2 tablespoons of oil or ghee in a large cast iron pan over medium heat. Drop heaping tablespoons of crab cake mixture into pan and gently press tops of mounds to shape into round cakes. Cook for 3–4 minutes or until a dark golden brown before carefully flipping and cooking for another 3 minutes. Place cooked crab cakes on a plate with paper towel.

To make remoulade mix minced cornichons with mayonnaise and Old Bay Seasoning.

Serve crab cakes with a dollop of remoulade and a sprinkling of minced parsley or chives.

# garlic-infused olive oil

**MAKES ½ CUP** | LF | V | GF

An easy way to make a mild olive oil that works well in salad dressings or to top steamed vegetables.

### INGREDIENTS

½ cup extra virgin olive oil

½ head garlic, separated into cloves, skins peeled, and woody ends removed

### PREPARATION

Pour one-third of the olive oil into a small saucepan. Heat over medium-low heat and toast garlic for 5 minutes until edges are a tiny bit golden. If it is browning too fast turn down heat. Add remaining oil and heat until edges of garlic are bubbling. Reduce to low and cook for 20 minutes. Allow to cool and strain through fine sieve. Make sure no garlic bits or skins remain—which can make oil go rancid quickly—and pour into a clean jar. Store in the refrigerator.

I like to make this in smaller batches so it keeps safely for a week. If you go through it quickly feel free to make larger batches.

Garlic-infused olive oil is an excellent alternative for those who love the flavor of garlic but can't tolerate straight garlic due to the fructans. Because fructans are water-soluble, they do not travel into the oil, giving you all the flavor with none of the upset.

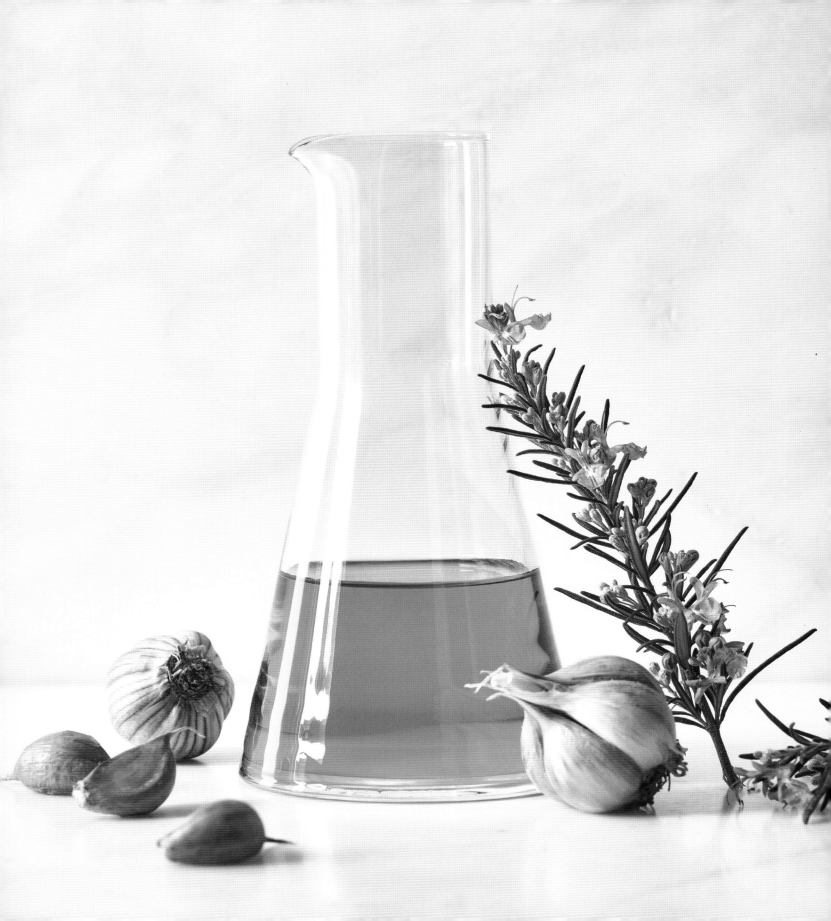

# carrot jicama slaw

**MAKES 3 CUPS** | LF | V | GF

This makes a great topping for salmon burgers or Pulled Pork (p. 140) sliders. And it makes a healthy main dish topped with lemongrass chicken, or steamed or grilled fish or shrimp.

### INGREDIENTS

3 carrots, grated or julienned

½ small jicama, grated or julienned

1 bunch cilantro, chopped

1 bunch mint, chiffonaded

Handful sesame seeds, and/or chopped peanuts, toasted

ginger + soy dipping sauce with a few drops of sesame oil added.

### PREPARATION

Toss vegetables, herbs, and dressing in a medium bowl. Season to taste and top with sesame seeds and/or peanuts

# asian-style cucumber salad

**MAKES 3 CUPS** | LF | V | GF

Crisp and cool, and very tasty, this salad complements almost any meal.

### INGREDIENTS

3 English cucumbers or six small Israeli cucumbers, cut into quarters lengthwise and sliced into ¼" slices

3 scallions, sliced thinly

2 tablespoons sesame seeds, toasted

2 tablespoons rice vinegar

1 tablespoon white wine vinegar

3 tablespoons coconut aminos or low sodium soy sauce

10 drops sesame oil

1 teaspoon dry mustard powder

Pinch chili flakes or more to taste

### PREPARATION

Combine all ingredients in a medium bowl and toss. Let marinate in dressing for 1 hour before serving

# herbed bread crumbs

**MAKES 1 CUP** | LF | V | GF

These are great to add a little crunch to almost anything—pasta, seafood, salads, etc. Small touches like these add a little excitement to the everyday.

### INGREDIENTS

3 tablespoons ghee

1 cup bread crumbs or almonds chopped finely in a food processor

1 teaspoon paprika

2 teaspoon dried herbs (I like a fine herb mix with chervil, tarragon, parsley, and chives)

1 clove of garlic, minced (optional)

### PREPARATION

Heat ghee in a small sauté pan, when melted add all ingredients and toast until crispy and golden. If using for a baked dish, like the Mac & Cheese, toast the bread crumbs for less time as they will continue to brown in the oven as a topping.

# salsa verde

**MAKES 1 ½ CUPS** | LF | V | GF

A vibrant, easy addition to your repertoire, this salsa brightens any meat dish and makes simple roasted vegetables more intriguing. Also, it's great on mashed potatoes. I have tried to cut corners by making it in the food processor, but trust me, it turns out much prettier if you take the time to hand chop those herbs. Plus washing, picking, and chopping the herbs can be a meditative task that smells good. Make sure they are dry before you chop them so they don't get mushy and brown. A salad spinner does the trick or you can just leave them to air dry for a few minutes on a clean kitchen towel.

### INGREDIENTS

1 bunch each, washed, dried, and finely chopped: parsley, tarragon, mint, and chives

½ teaspoon mustard seed, toasted and ground

½ teaspoon coriander, toasted and ground

½ teaspoon red chili flakes

Zest of 2 lemons

2 tablespoon red wine vinegar

1 tablespoon capers or 5 caper berries, finely chopped

1 teaspoon salt

Olive oil to cover (about 1 cup)

### PREPARATION

Mix all ingredients in a glass pint jar and cover with olive oil. Screw on the lid tightly and give it a good shake to mix it all together. Season to taste. It's better after it sits for a couple of hours. If refrigerating, leave out for an hour before serving so oil can liquefy.

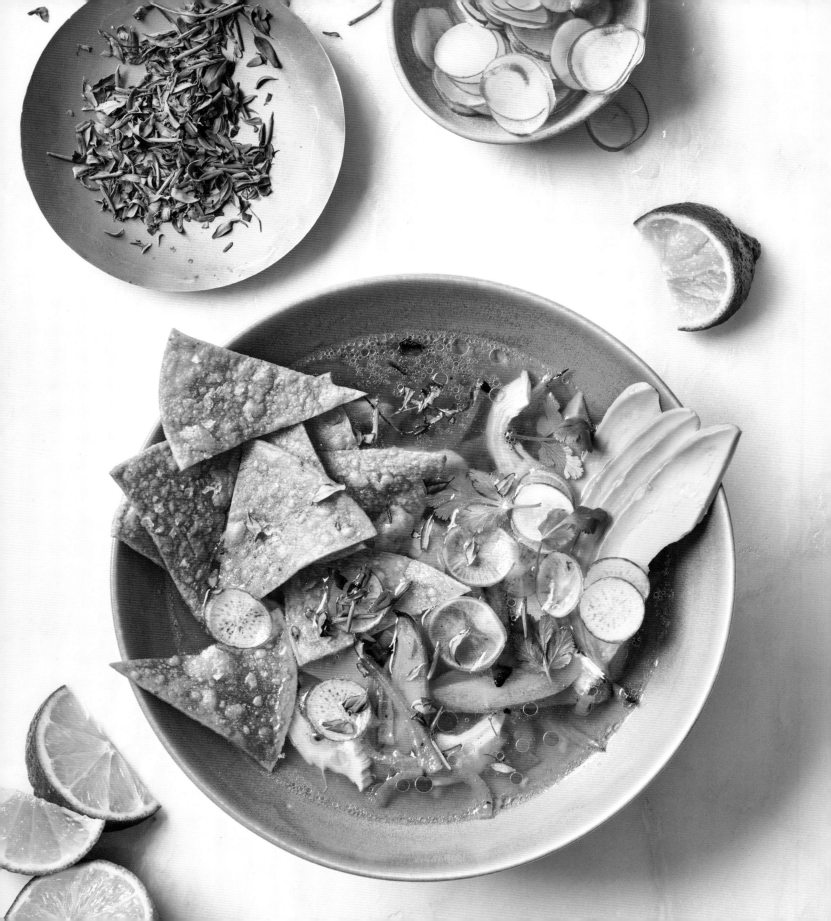

# chicken soup *with* variations

**MAKES 3 ½ QUARTS** | LF | V | GF

A whole chicken makes for a rich broth with perfectly cooked meat to add to your soup—a light, comforting meal all on its own or add a little something extra to a dinner. Blanching the chicken first keeps the broth pretty, clear, and clean tasting. It's a technique I use when making most meat broths. Roasting your vegetables in a super hot oven makes them flavorful without getting mushy. This basic recipe can be used as a stepping off point for many different variations.

## INGREDIENTS

**FOR THE BROTH:**

1 whole chicken cut into pieces, preferably pasture-raised

2 bay leaves

2 onions, halved

2 carrots, cut in large chunks

2 celery stalks, cut in large chunks

**TO FINISH SOUP:**

2 onions, cut into thin ¼ moons

2 carrots, sliced in ½ lengthwise and cut into ½ moons

2 stalks celery, thinly sliced

Olive oil

½ teaspoon coriander

½ teaspoon turmeric

1 tablespoon tomato paste

Salt

## PREPARATION

Preheat oven to broil. Place chicken in large pot. Cover with water and bring to a boil over high heat. Remove chicken pieces with tongs and discard water. Wash any foam from pot and put chicken back into pot. If stock is still cloudy repeat a second time.

Add vegetables for stock to chicken pieces and add just enough water to cover (about 3 quarts), add a few generous pinches of salt. Simmer on stovetop over low heat until chicken is falling off the bone (about 1–1½ hours), but be careful not to boil (boiling makes a cloudy broth).

While chicken is cooking, mix sliced vegetables with a generous drizzle of olive oil, coriander, turmeric, and a couple pinches of salt on a large parchment-lined sheet pan. Place under broiler, keeping a close eye on the vegetables. You want them to char around the edges but not to burn. Remove from oven and set aside once they are dark and crisp around the edges.

When chicken has cooked remove pieces from pot with tongs and let cool. Strain stock through cheesecloth and discard solids. Add tomato paste to broth and season to taste with desired flavorings.

When chicken is cool enough to handle, discard skin and pick meat from bones. You can keep bones in a container in the freezer for use in broth another time.

If serving in individual bowls, divide chicken and vegetables between bowls and ladle hot broth over the top. Or, mix chicken and vegetables together in a pot for people to serve themselves.

## VARIATIONS:

**For Mediterranean-style chicken soup garnish with:** Handful of fresh chopped oregano, thyme and/or dill, juice and zest of 1 lemon, fresh cracked black pepper

**For Asian-style soup:** Substitute kaffir lime leaf for bay leaf, then garnish with: ½ pound shiitake mushrooms, sliced and sautéed; 2 garlic cloves, sliced and sautéed; 1" piece of ginger, grated; cilantro, leaves picked off stems; juice and zest of 1 lime; coconut aminos and Asian chili paste to taste

**For chicken tortilla soup garnish with:** Juice and zest of 1 lime; chipotle chili paste from a can of chili in adobo, to taste; avocado, cut into cubes; jalapeño peppers, diced; oregano, chopped; good quality tortilla chips or homemade Baked Tortilla Chips (added at table)

# bone broth

**MAKES 3 QUARTS** | LF | GF

For chicken broth, a combination of chicken backs, necks, and feet work well. For beef broth, use marrow bones cut into pieces by your butcher. When you make a broth, note that anything the animal consumed (like antibiotics) is concentrated in the bones, so it's important to use the highest quality bones you can— organic/pasture-raised chicken and pork, grass-fed beef. The bones of well raised animals will produce a broth with a higher gelatin content, an indication the animals were raised in a humane environment.

## INGREDIENTS

3 pounds bones

3–4 quarts water

2 carrots

2 yellow onions

2 stalks celery

½ bunch parsley (omit for pregnant or breastfeeding women)

1 tablespoon peppercorns

2 bay leaves

10 stems thyme

1 tablespoon wine or rice vinegar

## PREPARATION

Preheat oven to 425°F (220°C). Place bones in a large stockpot and cover with cold water, bring to a boil then simmer for 20 minutes. Strain off water and rinse bones. This eliminates any impurities and keeps your broth from having an off flavor. I have skipped this step with chicken bones and it turned out fine, no funky flavors, nothing was ruined by not blanching. That said, this step will ensure your chicken stock is clear and should never, never be skipped with beef and pork bone. It is a very sad moment when you have been cooking your broth for 24 hours to discover it doesn't taste right because the bones weren't blanched.

Cover a large sheet pan with parchment and spread bones in a single layer. Roast at 425°F (220°C) for about 1 hour. You want the bones deeply roasted, they should be a nice, dark brown. This will give you a rich broth without having to add many other ingredients. For chicken broth, if you are looking for a light, mild broth you can skip this step. But both beef and pork bones need roasting.

Put roasted bones along with any brown bits from the roasting pan back in your large, now clean, stockpot. Carefully pour the rendered fat that is pooling in the bottom of the pan into a clean jar and freeze for later use.

*There's rarely a week that goes by that we don't enjoy a broth in some form, either as a base to a soup, a liquid for rice, or just on its own. Technically, broths can be cooked for two hours, but we keep ours on a slow simmer for many hours (ideally 24) to pull out as much collagen as possible. Light but rich with flavor, broths are filled with a wealth of nutritional benefits.*

---

- They are a potent source of essential minerals and electrolytes: calcium, magnesium, and phosphorous.

- They are hydrating and support electrolyte balance.

- They are full of various amino acids, which are the building blocks for proteins in the body and essential for healthy growth and metabolism.

- They serve various functions within the body, reducing inflammation and boosting immunity.

- When SIBO or other gut issues make us feel out of balance, broths are a wonderfully mild way to hydrate and ingest a small boost of protein, giving our systems a bit of fuel without further upset.

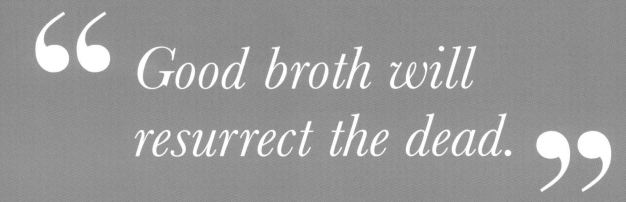

## " *Good broth will resurrect the dead.* "

# french onion soup

**MAKES 1 ½–2 QUARTS** | LF | V | GF

Onions are not only super flavorful, they are rich in antioxidants and they assist the liver in eliminating toxins. They are transformed into sweet and earthy deliciousness by slow caramelization. This soup is so satisfying you'll want to make it again and again.

## INGREDIENTS

4 tablespoons of butter

2 yellow onions, sliced thinly

2 red onions, sliced thinly

4 shallots, sliced thinly

2 tablespoons Dijon mustard

2 tablespoons thyme, chopped

Handful of parsley, finely chopped, and 1 tablespoon reserved for garnish

Splash of white wine, sherry, or vermouth

5 cups beef, chicken, or vegetable broth + more if needed to thin soup to desired consistency

2 tablespoons coconut aminos

1 teaspoon high fructose-free Worcestershire Sauce or another teaspoon of coconut aminos

Salt and ground black pepper, to taste

2 cups Gruyère cheese, grated

6 thick slices of sourdough

## PREPARATION

Preheat oven to 350°F (180°C). In a large pan, caramelize onions with 4 tablespoons of butter and a pinch of salt for 45 minutes over low heat until soft and golden brown. Stir mustard, thyme, parsley, and another pinch of salt into the onions and cook over medium heat for 2 minutes. Deglaze pan with a splash of sherry or white wine. Cook for another 2 minutes or until alcohol smell cooks out.

Add all other ingredients and let simmer for an additional 30 minutes, adding salt, pepper, and additional Worcestershire Sauce (or coconut aminos), to taste, after the first 15 minutes of simmering.

When soup is almost done simmering, lay sourdough slices on a parchment-lined sheet pan and cover each with cheese. Bake for 15 minutes or until cheese is melted and golden.

Ladle soup into bowls and top with bread and remaining parsley.

# potato, leek & mushroom soup

**MAKES 2 ½ QUARTS** | LF | V | GF

Creamy, comforting, and dairy-free goodness—a lighter version of cream of your typical mushroom soup. Seasoning through each step of the process ensures a well-rounded flavor.

### INGREDIENTS

4 tablespoons butter, ghee, or olive oil

2 leeks, chopped

3 cloves garlic, chopped

2 pounds cremini mushrooms, roughly chopped

6 mushrooms reserved and sliced thin for garnish

3 tablespoons thyme, chopped

1 quart chicken stock or vegetable stock + 2 cups to adjust thickness if needed

3 large potatoes, peeled and cut in 1" cubes, about 4 cups (any type of potato will do)

1 Parmesan rind (optional, but recommended)

Juice of ½ lemon + more to taste, if needed

Salt

Chives, chopped for garnish

### PREPARATION

In a large soup pot, heat the butter over medium heat. Add the leeks and two generous pinches of salt. Cook about 10 minutes, stirring occasionally, until leeks are very tender. Add the garlic and sauté another 30 seconds.

Add the mushrooms, thyme, and another pinch of salt. Stir and cook 15 minutes until mushrooms start to brown.

Add the stock, potatoes, and Parmesan rind. Bring to a boil, reduce to a simmer, and cook uncovered for 30–40 minutes, until potatoes and mushrooms are tender. Taste and add salt as needed. Remove the Parmesan rind and discard.

Working in batches, transfer the soup to a blender and mix until smooth or using a stick blender to blend in pot. Adjust seasoning to taste, add salt and lemon juice as needed. Add broth to desired consistency

In a sauté pan, heat 1 teaspoon olive oil and sauté the thinly sliced mushrooms until tender, along with a pinch of salt.

Ladle the soup into bowls and garnish with chopped chives and sautéed mushrooms.

# bolognese

**MAKES 1 QUART** | LF | GF

For this hearty and rich recipe, it's worth it to make sure to buy high-quality, humanely-raised meat. You can substitute chopped leftover roast beef or pot roast for part of the ground meat. Using a sauce made from fresh tomatoes rather than canned tomatoes cuts cooking time in half, but both taste great.

## INGREDIENTS

¼ pound preservative-free pancetta

Olive oil

1 onion

2 carrots, diced

2 celery stalks, diced

¼ pound free-range or pasture-raised ground turkey

¼ pound grass-fed ground beef

¼ pound pasture-raised ground pork

Handful of oregano, minced

Handful of parsley, minced

Handful of thyme, minced

5 sage leaves, minced

10 basil leaves, chiffonaded

1 cup dry white wine

3 cups Simple Summertime Tomato Sauce (p. 79) or 1 large can diced tomatoes

4 cups beef, chicken, or vegetable broth

Salt and ground black pepper, to taste

## PREPARATION

In a large saucepan over medium heat, sauté pancetta until lightly golden. Add olive oil if needed and add vegetables, cook for 15–20 minutes. When nicely browned, add ground meat along with half of the chopped herbs. Season generously with salt and pepper and cook, breaking into small pieces until browned, about 20 minutes more.

Add white wine, scraping brown bits from bottom of pan. Add tomatoes and reduce heat to medium-low. Add broth and a couple pinches of salt and cook for 3 hours, stirring every so often and adding more water or broth if needed.

In last 30 minutes of cooking, add remaining herbs and season to taste. When finished, the tomatoes should be a deep red and the fat will be separated on top of sauce. If you would like a more homogeneous sauce you can use a stick blender and pulse for a few seconds to bring sauce together.

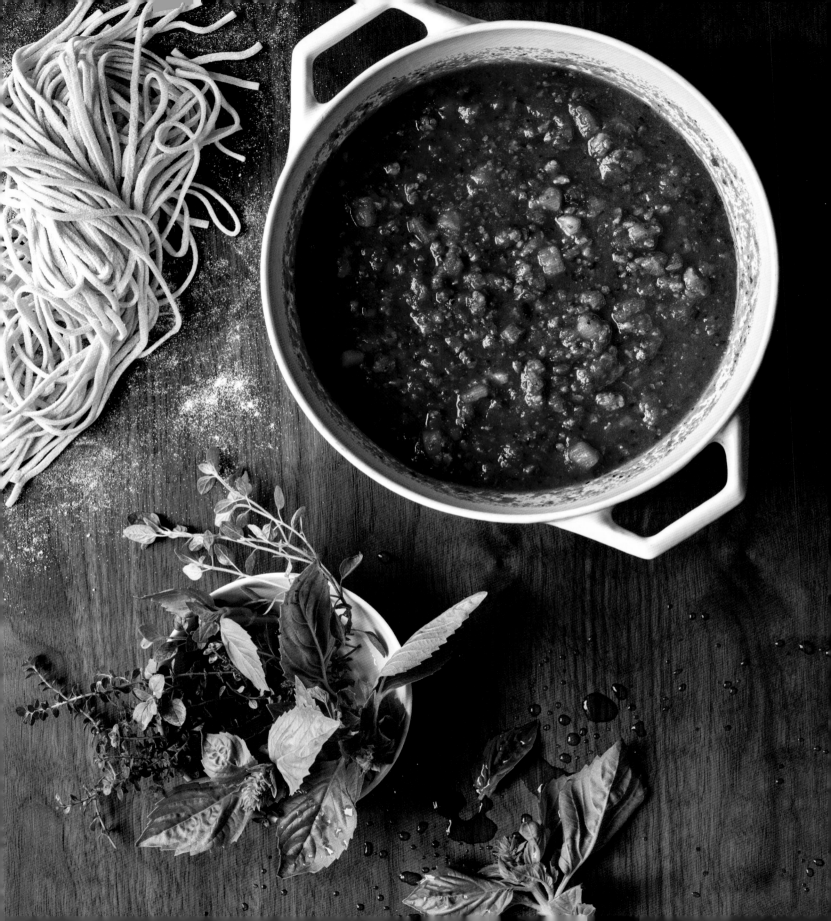

# spaghetti *with* turkey meatballs

**MAKES 18 MEATBALLS** | LF

Here's a comforting meal for chilly weather or for a cozy weekend dinner. The spinach, cheese, and panko prevent the dry turkey meatball downfall. Cooking a test spoonful of the meatball mixture ensures your meatballs are flavorful and seasoned to your liking.

## INGREDIENTS

### MEATBALLS:

1½ pounds ground dark meat turkey

2 eggs, whisked

1 bunch spinach, sautéed, water pressed out and finely chopped

⅓ cup panko bread crumbs

1 cup Parmesan cheese, finely grated

1 bunch sage, minced

½ bunch parsley, minced

½ bunch thyme, minced

1 tablespoon garlic, minced

1 tablespoon dried basil

1 tablespoon fennel seeds, toasted and ground

1 tablespoon minced dried onion

Pinch cayenne pepper

½ teaspoon ground black pepper

1 teaspoon salt

### SAUCE:

3 cups Simple Summertime Tomato Sauce (p. 79) or 1 large can diced tomatoes

½ cup dry red or white wine

Olive oil

## PREPARATION

In a large mixing bowl, combine all ingredients except tomatoes, wine, and olive oil. Heat a small amount of oil in a large Dutch oven and cook a small spoonful of meat mixture. Taste and adjust seasoning as needed. Repeat if necessary.

When mixture is seasoned, heat another couple tablespoons of olive oil in Dutch oven over low heat. Roll into 1½" balls and place into hot pan. Using tongs, gently turn meatballs so that they brown on all sides. When meatballs are evenly browned, pour tomatoes over top along with ½ cup wine.

Simmer over medium-low heat for 45 minutes until sauce reduces and meatballs are fully cooked. Season to taste and serve with spaghetti or your favorite vegetable noodle substitute.

# gnocchi

**MAKES 4–6 SERVINGS** | LF | V | GF
Adapted from *Smitten Kitchen*

An easy pasta to make, these are great tossed with brown butter and sage, or pesto or tomato sauces. They can also be cooked and dropped into tomato soup as dumplings.

## INGREDIENTS

2 pounds russet potatoes, scrubbed

1 egg and 1 teaspoon of salt, beaten with a fork

1½ cups flour

## PREPARATION

Preheat oven to 350°F (180°C). Poke potatoes with a fork and place in a baking dish covered with foil. Bake for 1–1½ hours until a butter knife slides through effortlessly.

After baking let potatoes cool, covered, for 15 minutes or until they are cool enough to handle. Pull skins off along with any parts of the potato that might have browned in the oven and grate through the small holes of a cheese grater. They will be crumbly so make sure to break up any larger pieces that crumble before being grated.

Pour egg and salt mixture over potatoes and mix thoroughly with a wooden spoon. Add the flour a ½ cup at a time until the dough holds together and becomes smooth and easy to work with.

Turn dough out onto a floured surface and knead for 5 minutes to form a uniform dough.

Divide dough into 6 balls and roll each into a 1" rope. Cut into ¾" pieces.

To cook, carefully drop the pieces into a pot of salted boiling water. After 2 or 3 minutes they will start to float to the top and can be scooped out with a slotted spoon and tossed in whatever sauce you like.

# traditional mac & cheese

**SERVES 6–8** | LF | V

This is a lovely mac and cheese to make and serve right out of the pot and topped with extra crispy crumbs. Made with a roux, it is thick and creamy. However, it can get a little grainy when reheating so we prefer to eat it right away.

## INGREDIENTS

1 pound cavatappi pasta, cooked and tossed with ghee while making sauce (leave in pasta pot)

3 tablespoon ghee

3 tablespoons flour

4 cups lactose-free whole milk or almond milk (use the highest quality almond milk you can find without fillers or gums)

1 pound Gruyère cheese, grated

½ pound Parmesan cheese, grated

1 teaspoon dry yellow mustard, ground

½ teaspoon nutmeg

1 teaspoon salt + more for pasta water and to taste

Herbed Bread Crumbs (p. 175), toasted to be extra toasty

## PREPARATION

Over medium-low heat melt ghee in large saucepan, add flour and cook until flour is a very light brown and smells nutty. Add milk cup by cup whisking between additions. It will become very thick at first and then get watery as you add more milk. When all the milk is added and there are no lumps, add cheese by the handful, whisking and making sure each addition is fully melted and incorporated before adding another handful. Make sure the mixture never reaches a full simmer.

When all the cheese is added, season with mustard, nutmeg, and salt. Let cook over low heat until mixture is thick and creamy. Warm pasta, pour cheese sauce over top of pasta in the pasta pot and mix thoroughly. Move pasta and sauce mixture into serving bowl and top with bread crumbs. Serve immediately.

# super gooey scientific mac & cheese

**SERVES 6–8** | LF | V | GF

When we first started out with our traditional mac and cheese recipe we thought it was delicious—rich and flavorful with a toasty bread crumb topping. But we wanted something that didn't get grainy when refrigerated. I had recently come across an incredibly informative article in *Cooks Illustrated* about using sodium citrate as a way to make a quick, easy, super creamy and smooth mac and cheese, so we thought we would order some online and give it a try. Sodium citrate is a natural salt derived from citrus, and sparing you all the molecular biology details, it breaks down the cheese in a way that leaves you with an incredibly silky sauce that reheats like a dream. You have to order it online as it is a specialty item not found on the shelves of your regular grocery store.

We added more Parmesan, because by omitting butter and flour, it helps to mellow out the flavors. More Gruyère makes for a very adult mac and cheese, which we liked, but the kids didn't. Play with ratios as you please, just make sure you have 2 pounds of cheese total. And, because the sauce doesn't include flour, you can simply use gluten-free pasta and bread crumbs to make a gluten-free mac and cheese if you like.

## INGREDIENTS

1 pound cavatappi pasta, cooked and tossed with ghee while making sauce (leave in pasta pot)

4 teaspoons sodium citrate

3 cups lactose-free milk or water, or almond milk (use the highest quality almond milk you can find without fillers or gums)

½ pound Gruyère cheese, grated

1½ pound Parmesan cheese, grated

1 teaspoon dry yellow mustard, ground

½ teaspoon white pepper

½ teaspoon nutmeg

1 teaspoon salt + more for pasta water and to taste

Herbed Bread Crumbs (p. 175)

## PREPARATION

In large saucepan over low heat combine sodium citrate with whatever liquid you are using, whisk until dissolved. Add cheese handful by handful and blend with a hand blender after each addition making sure each addition is fully melted and incorporated before adding another handful. When all cheese is melted, add spices and blend as necessary until sauce is completely smooth. Season sauce to taste.

Pour sauce over pasta and mix thoroughly. Move onto greased baking dish and top with bread crumbs. This can be refrigerated for up to five days and will last, if well wrapped, for at least a month in the freezer.

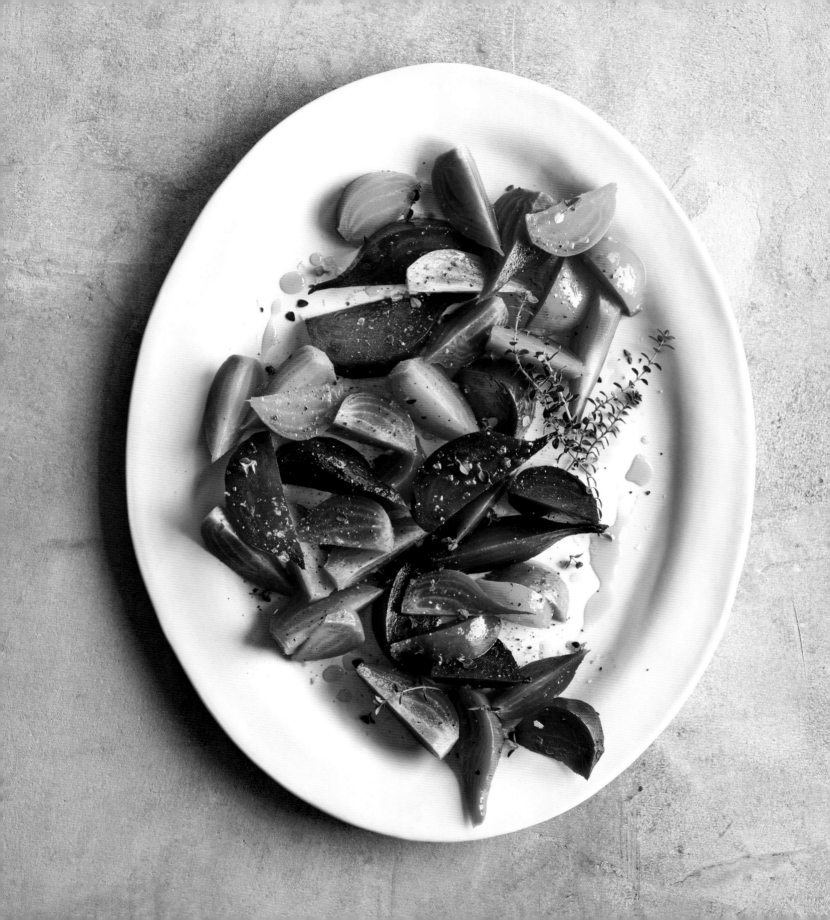

# easy citrus marinated beets

**SERVES 6–8** | LF | V | GF

The citrus pairs well with the earthiness of the beets. This recipe adds a light touch to a meal even in the dead of winter, especially when the vegetable selection on the East Coast looks a little sad. Also perfect for a summer picnic or out of the container as a midnight snack. I usually cook one large beet per person so feel free to adjust amounts if you are on your own or cooking for a big group of friends.

## INGREDIENTS

6 beets

Water

¼ cup rice vinegar + a splash to finish

Few sprigs of thyme and parsley
+ 1 tablespoon each, minced

Juice of 2 oranges

Zest of 1 lemon

Salt and ground black pepper, to taste

## PREPARATION

Preheat oven to 350°F (180°C). Put beets in a shallow saucepan with a lid. Add enough water to pan so that water comes halfway up the side of the beets. Add ¼ cup vinegar, a generous sprinkle of salt, and whole herb sprigs. Cover and bake until a butter knife easily slides through the middle of the largest beet, about 45 minutes to 1 hour. When tender, let cool in covered pot until cool enough to handle. Peel and cut into quarters. Toss with juice from oranges, lemon zest, herbs, a couple big pinches of salt, and a splash of vinegar. Refrigerate and season with vinegar, salt and pepper to taste before serving.

# green beans *with* toasted nuts

**SERVES 6–8** | LF | V | GF

Giving the green beans a little bit of steam at the start get them perfectly tender before finishing them in oil on high heat. Pecans are my favorite nuts to use, but feel free to top the beans with any nuts you have on hand. Macadamia nuts are fun, almonds are classic, peanuts give a little Asian flair and go well with a few chili flakes and ginger.

**INGREDIENTS**

2½ pounds green beans, ends trimmed

2 tablespoons olive oil

3 cloves garlic, sliced thinly

Juice of ½ lemon

Salt

Crumbled pecans, toasted

**PREPARATION**

Over high heat, add green beans to extra large pan with two tablespoons of water and a generous pinch of salt—make two batches if your pan is on the small side. Cover for 3 minutes and allow to steam. Remove lid and let water evaporate, about 1 minute. When the water has evaporated add oil. Stirring only occasionally, allow the green beans to sear slightly. When beans are just about done add garlic and cook until garlic is toasted and beans are al dente. Toss with lemon juice and top with toasted nuts and crunchy salt.

You can also add 1 tablespoon balsamic vinegar once you add the olive oil and let it cook down to make balsamic glazed green beans.

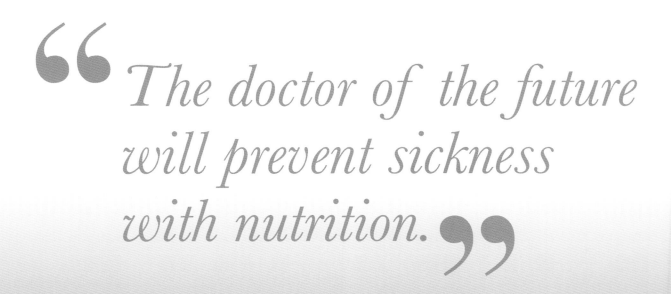

*" The doctor of the future will prevent sickness with nutrition. "*

# weeknight risotto

**MAKES 7 CUPS** | LF | V | GF

Risotto is one of those dishes that can seem intimidating but can easily becomes a regular weeknight side dish. No need to stir constantly; just after every ladleful of stock and then every couple of minutes to make sure the rice doesn't stick to the bottom of the pan. Gradually adding the stock helps the rice cook evenly, staying creamy without being mushy.

Once you are comfortable with the basic recipe you can experiment with different variations. When adding other ingredients, like roasted vegetables, add them right before the last addition of stock so the flavor incorporates with the rice but vegetables don't disintegrate. Vegetables should be fully cooked but still a little al dente before adding to rice.

## INGREDIENTS

1 onion, diced

2 celery stalks, diced

2¼ cups arborio or carnaroli rice

½ cup white wine (optional)

¼ teaspoon saffron, add to stock while it is heating

1 tablespoon thyme, chopped

2 tablespoons ghee or olive oil

8 cups broth, keep hot in saucepan

1 cup Parmesan cheese, grated

Salt and ground black pepper, to taste

## PREPARATION

In a medium saucepan over medium-high heat, sauté vegetables in olive oil (or ghee) with a couple pinches of salt until golden. Add rice and cook for a few minutes until the rice is coated in olive oil and slightly translucent. Add wine if using and stir until it is evaporated. Reduce heat to medium-low and add hot stock by the ladleful, about 1 cup at a time. Stir until rice is coated then stir every couple of minutes until stock is absorbed. If rice is sticking, lower heat. Keep adding stock. When approximately ¾ of the stock is used, taste and season with salt. At this point the rice should be getting soft. Taste after next few additions to make sure rice isn't getting mushy. Rice should be creamy at the end. Add herbs and grated cheese and season to taste.

## VARIATIONS:

Replace half the broth with butternut squash soup and add diced, roasted squash and chopped fresh sage. Top with fried sage leaves.

Use mushroom stock, add sautéed mushrooms and swap out the Parmesan for Gruyère.

Use half fish stock and half fresh tomato sauce, add zucchini, lemon zest, and a squeeze of lemon juice before your last addition of broth. Top with grilled shrimp

# skirt steak *with* salsa verde

**SERVES 6–8** | LF | GF

Try this for a super quick weeknight dinner. Skirt steak is a tender, flavorful cut of beef and is simple to cook. It needs only salt, pepper, and a very hot pan—just a few minutes on each side to reach a juicy medium rare. Skirt steak is its most tender when cooked medium rare, so if needed, use a meat thermometer to ensure it doesn't overcook. Slice against the grain for optimum tenderness. Also skirt steak is a great cut for steak tacos, fajitas, and stir-fry recipes.

### INGREDIENTS

2½ pounds skirt steak (grass-fed), cut in half or quarters if needed to fit in pan

Salt and ground black pepper, to taste

Salsa Verde (p. 175)

### PREPARATION

Liberally season both sides of the steaks with salt and pepper, about ¼ teaspoon of salt and ten grinds of fresh pepper per side. Preheat a heavy skillet or cast iron pan until very hot, about 4 minutes over high heat. When pan is hot, lay steaks in pan and cook on each side for 3–4 minutes until medium rare. Let rest for 5 minutes before cutting steak into slices—lengthwise against grain. Top with Salsa Verde and crunchy salt to finish.

You can also cook on a grill. Just make sure your grill is very hot before cooking.

## NOT ALL BEEF IS CREATED EQUALLY AND WHY THAT MATTERS TO YOUR GUT HEALTH

Red meat is always a media darling, both fetishized (can you say Kobe?) and demonized. We firmly believe it can be a wonderfully nutritious addition to a diet, but quality is key. We recommend spending a bit more for 100% grass-fed, even if it means eating a bit less of it. Grass-fed beef—the diet a cow is designed to eat—is higher in key nutrients, antioxidants, vitamins and CLA (a beneficial fat that has been linked to improved immunity and anti-inflammatory benefits), and is much less likely to contain antibiotic "superbugs." It's also not great for microbiome-diversity: a nationwide study of corn-fed chicken showed almost the exact same chemical composition of their meat in every sample, less diversity than would be found in grass-fed animals raised in just one farmyard.

# chicken tagine *with* preserved lemons *&* olives

**SERVES 6–8** LF | V | GF

This can be made in a traditional tagine or Dutch oven for a light, bright dish. A tagine can only be used over medium-low heat, so it's important to sear the chicken in a separate skillet to build flavor and give the chicken a beautiful golden color. We love this with saffron and almond couscous or rice. Preserved lemons can be found at most high-end and Middle Eastern grocery stores (sometimes they are called pickled lemons).

## INGREDIENTS

1 whole chicken, cut into pieces or 10 chicken thighs

1 tablespoon salt

1 tablespoon ground ginger

2 teaspoons cinnamon

2 teaspoons ground coriander

2 teaspoons turmeric

2 tablespoons ghee

4 red onions, thinly sliced lengthwise

1 tablespoon honey

6 garlic cloves, sliced

Juice of 1 lemon

1½ cups oil-cured or Kalamata olives, pitted and halved

1 bunch cilantro, roughly chopped

1 cup chicken broth

4 preserved lemons, roughly chopped

Salt and ground black pepper, to taste

## PREPARATION

Toss chicken with salt and spices, cover and let sit for 1 hour or refrigerate overnight.

Preheat oven to 350°F (180°C). Add ghee to Dutch oven or large skillet (if you will be braising in a tagine) over medium-high heat and sear chicken pieces until skin is brown and crispy. Remove from pan and set aside. Add onions to pan with honey and caramelize for 30 minutes with a couple generous pinches of salt. Add garlic for last 5 minutes of caramelizing onions.

When onions are golden and soft, deglaze pan with lemon juice scraping up brown bits. Toss onion and lemon mixture with half of the chopped cilantro and broth. Top with chicken pieces. If you are baking in a tagine, transfer onions to tagine to assemble. Nestle olives, garlic, and preserved lemons around chicken. Season with pepper and place covered pot in oven and bake for 45 minutes to 1 hour, until chicken is cooked through. If cooking in a Dutch oven, cook uncovered for last 15 minutes of cooking so that sauce can thicken.

Top with remaining cilantro and season to taste with lemon juice, salt and pepper.

# whole roasted chicken

**SERVES 4–6** | LF | GF

Serve this for a weeknight one-pan meal. Salting the chicken and letting it rest gives it a crispy skin and adds flavor. Starting the roast breast side down keeps the breast meat from drying out. We sometimes roast two chickens at a time to serve six with enough leftovers to add to salads and sandwiches and sautéed with chopped onions for last-minute chicken tacos.

## INGREDIENTS

1 whole, pasture raised chicken, 4–6 pounds

1 tablespoon salt

Handful of sage leaves, chopped

1 tablespoon thyme, chopped

½ tablespoon paprika

Ground black pepper

3 carrots, cut into 1" pieces

3 celery stalks, cut into 1" pieces

3 potatoes, cut into 1" pieces

1 red onion, cut 1" pieces

Head of garlic, cloves separated and peeled

Olive oil

1 lemon, cut in half

A few whole thyme and sage sprigs

## PREPARATION

Season chicken inside and out with salt, herbs, paprika, and pepper. Refrigerate overnight or let sit at room temperature for 1 hour. If refrigerating, let rest at room temperature for 1 hour before roasting.

Preheat oven to 400°F (200°C). Place vegetables and half of the garlic in bottom of roasting pan, toss with a light coating of olive oil and season with a few large pinches of salt and pepper. Place lemon halves, the remaining half of garlic, and herb sprigs inside of the chicken then roast breast side down for 45 minutes. Flip chicken so breast side is up and roast for another 20–30 minutes until skin is crisp and thigh meat is no longer pink and juices run clear.

# fish cooked *in* parchment

**SERVES 4-6** | LF | GF

This is my go-to for an easy weeknight dinner or dinner party. The fish stays moist and the variations are endless. It's nutritious and easy, and each packet can be a full meal by laying fish on a bed of thinly sliced vegetables and topping with whatever herbs and spices you like. Plan for about 1 cup of vegetables per person. I usually make a little extra to have leftovers to add to salads or sandwiches for an easy lunch the next day.

## INGREDIENT IDEAS

### THAI:

Cod on a bed of thinly sliced red bell peppers and green beans topped with kaffir lime leaf, two tablespoons coconut milk, coconut aminos, and a squeeze of lime juice.

### MEDITERRANEAN:

Wild caught salmon on a bed of zucchini, fennel, and red onions tossed with salt and olive oil then topped with a few sprigs of fresh thyme, halved cherry tomatoes, and a splash of white wine. Slice zucchini, fennel, and red onions as thinly as possible (or a mandoline works great for this).

### ITALIAN:

Halibut on a bed of chard (stems and leaves finely chopped) tossed with a pinch of salt and squeeze of lemon juice then topped with diced tomatoes, capers, Kalamata olives, thinly sliced garlic, and a drizzle of olive oil.

### CHINESE:

Sea bass on a bed of spinach tossed with a pinch of salt and thinly sliced scallions then topped with minced ginger, garlic, a squeeze of lime juice, and a teaspoon of coconut aminos or low sodium soy sauce.

## PREPARATION

A rule of thumb is 6–8 ounces of fish per person. Have the fishmonger remove the skin or slice off before cooking—steamed fish skin isn't very tasty. I love the precut unbleached parchment sheets, but any parchment paper cut into roughly 12 × 16" rectangles works well. Lay all of the ingredients in the middle of the parchment and fold parchment over top. Starting at one edge of the parchment fold parchment together forming a crescent shaped package

Cook packets on a sheet pan at 400°F (200°C). Cooking times vary based on the size of the fillets you are using. For thin fillets like sole or char cook for 10–15 minutes, for thicker fillets like halibut or salmon cook for 15–20 minutes.

You can serve in individual packets—it's fun for people to open their own little present. You can also prepare a whole fillet in a larger packet, cook it for an extra 5–10 minutes and serve family style.

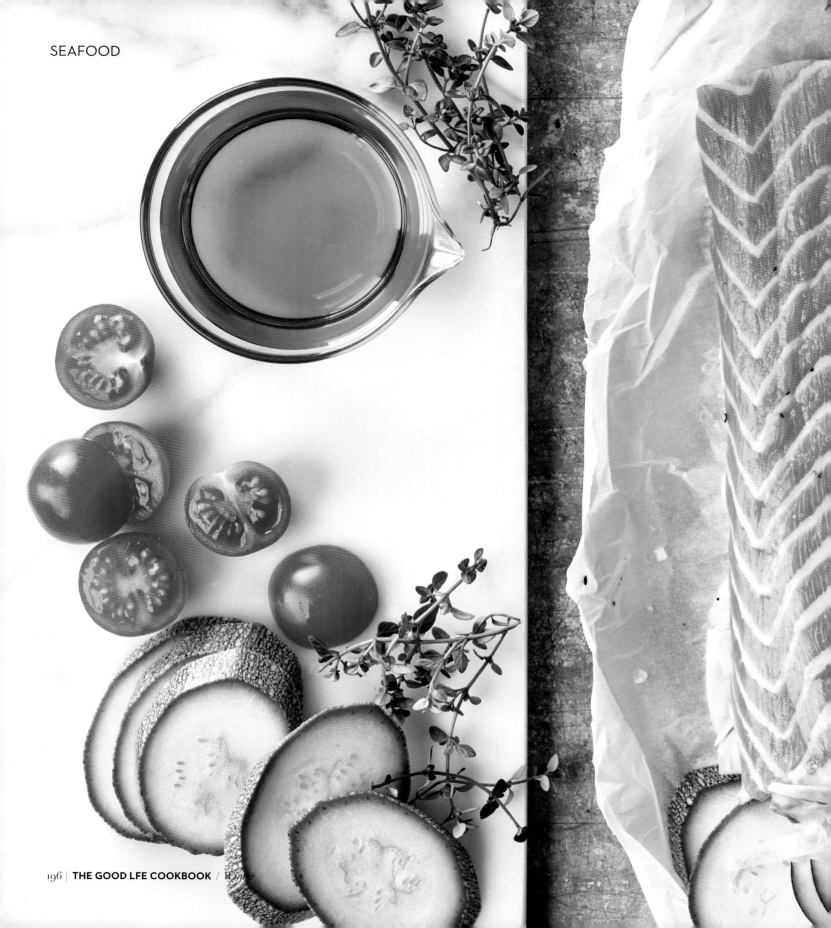

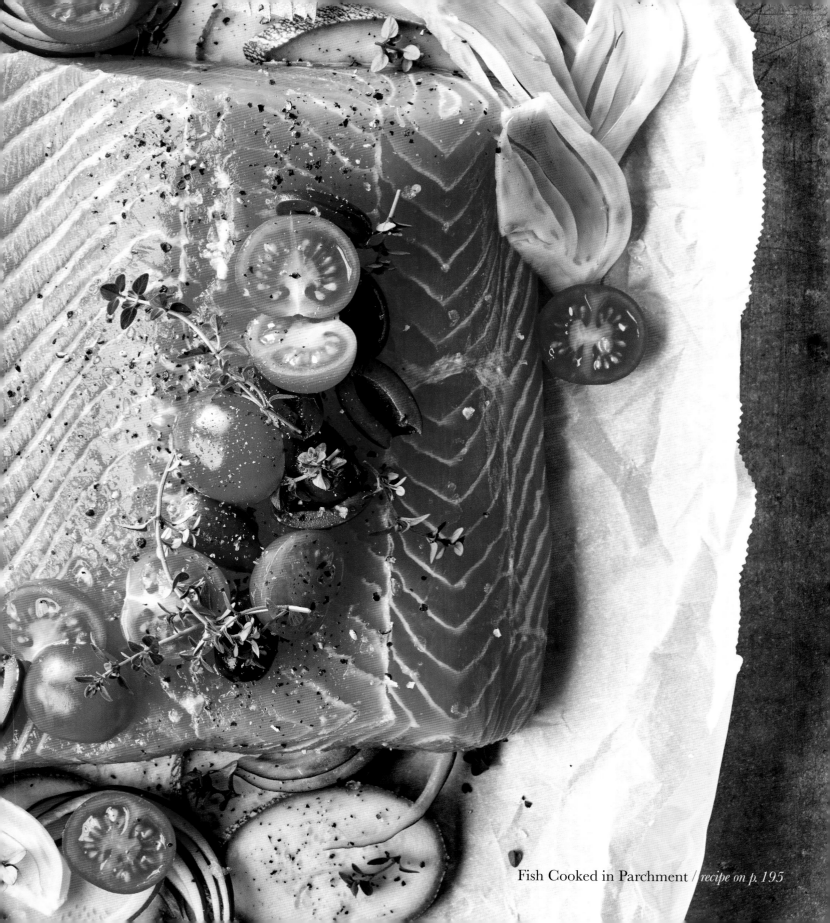

Fish Cooked in Parchment / *recipe on p. 195*

# panko-crusted fish

**MAKES 6 FILLETS** | LF | GF

Adapted from *Ina Garten's Barefoot Contessa: How Easy Is That*

Salmon is a great source of Omega-3 fatty acids. You can buy the whole fillet and cut the salmon into 6 servings to prepare recipe below or buy already cut pieces of salmon. Leftovers are great for salads.

## INGREDIENTS

2 pounds wild Alaskan salmon or arctic char

Salt and ground black pepper, to taste

2 tablespoons Dijon mustard

2 tablespoons ghee

1 cup Herbed Bread Crumbs (p. 175) mixed with:

3 tablespoons parsley, minced

Zest of 1 lemon

## PREPARATION

Preheat the oven to 425 degrees. Lightly sprinkle both sides of fish with salt and pepper.

Brush mustard on top of salmon. Heat oil over medium-high heat in a heavy 12" ovenproof pan. When the oil is hot, add the salmon skin side down, and sear for 4 minutes, without turning. You want the skin to brown but not burn. Remove pan from heat and press panko mixture on top of the mustard on the salmon creating a thick coating on top. Transfer the pan to the hot oven and bake for 6–8 minutes until the salmon is cooked through and the panko is browned. Remove from the oven very carefully. The pan is extremely hot.*

*Remember to always have an oven mitt or two holding the pan. It is so easy to forget how hot the pan is right out of the oven. Unfortunately, I have burned my hand a few times while making this dish.

# shrimp scampi

**SERVES 6–8** | LF | GF

Adapted from *Bon Appétit*

Shrimp scampi is one of those dishes you barely need a recipe for—I've been making it off the top of my head for decades. So when I came across the *Bon Appétit* recipe that called for marinating the shrimp before cooking, I was intrigued. I gave it a try and indeed it does add an extra layer of flavor. We modified it to be SIBO-friendly and added tarragon. I love tarragon with seafood, shrimp in particular. This can be served over pasta, spaghetti squash, rice, or with toasted crusty bread.

## INGREDIENTS

10 garlic cloves, 4 grated on microplane, 6 thinly sliced

Salt to taste

4 tablespoons olive oil, divided in half

3 pounds cleaned and deveined shrimp

1 teaspoon chili flakes

¾ cup dry white wine

Zest of 1 lemon

3 tablespoons cold ghee or butter

½ bunch parsley, minced, saving some for garnish

½ bunch tarragon, minced

1 tablespoon dried sumac

## PREPARATION

Toss microplaned garlic, 2 teaspoons of salt, and half the olive oil with the shrimp in a medium bowl. Cover and refrigerate for 1 hour.

Heat remaining olive oil in large skillet over low heat, add shrimp mixture and cook until shrimp are half cooked—about 2 minutes, turning shrimp halfway through. Remove shrimp from pan.

Cook sliced garlic and chili flakes for 1 minute, add wine and lemon zest and cook over medium heat until wine is reduced and no longer smells like alcohol, about 3 minutes. Whisk in ghee and continue whisking and cooking until sauce has thickened. Add shrimp back to pan along with herbs and sumac and cook for another 2 minutes. Transfer to serving bowl, toss with pasta if serving with pasta, and garnish with remaining parsley.

# fudge

**MAKES 25 (1 ½") SQUARES** | V | GF

Just a few ingredients are needed for this fudge. It's not too sweet, it's dairy-free and delicious, and SIBO-friendly!

## INGREDIENTS

1 can coconut milk

¼ cup sugar

3 cups chocolate chips (bittersweet or semisweet depending on how sweet you want it)

1½ cups toasted nuts and/or shredded coconut (optional)

Crunchy salt (optional)

## PREPARATION

Combine coconut milk and sugar in a small saucepan and cook over medium-low heat, stirring often, for 45 minutes or until coconut milk is reduced by half and coats the back of a spoon.

Combine 1 cup of your sweetened condensed coconut milk (reserve the rest for tea or spooning over berries) with chocolate chips in a mixing bowl and place on top of a double boiler over medium heat. Stir until chocolate is melted.

Combine with 1 cup nuts, if using, and pour into a small, parchment-lined 8" baking dish. Top with remaining nuts and salt.

Refrigerate until set, about 3 hours. Cut into 1½" squares. Store in airtight container in refrigerator or freezer until ready to eat.

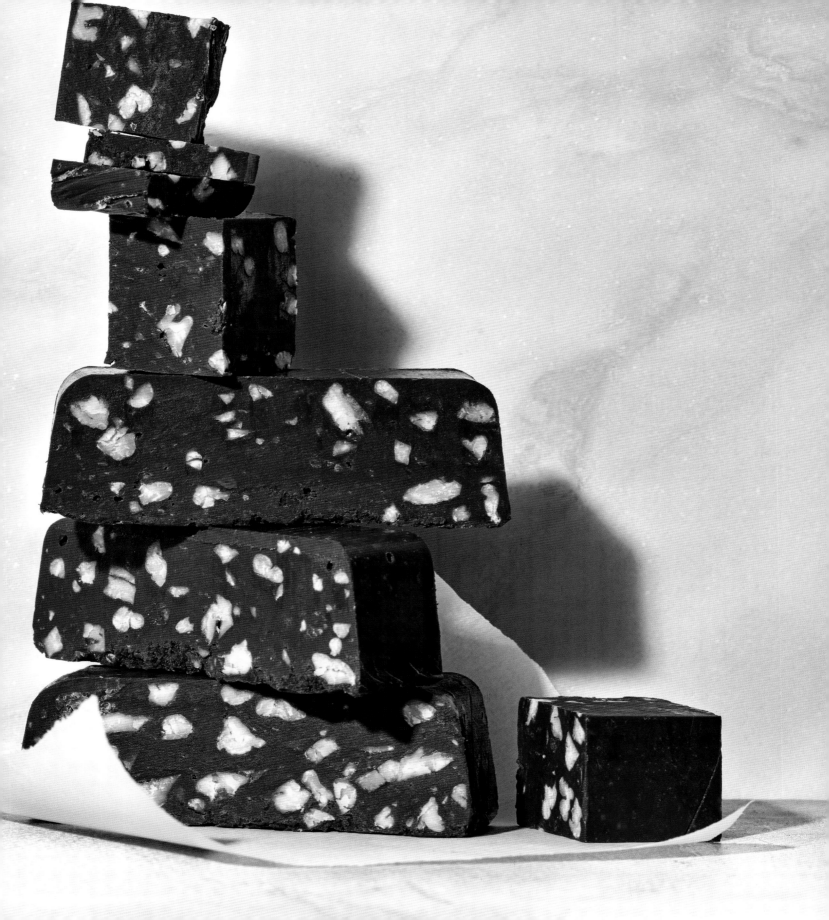

# pecan & cinnamon sticky buns

**MAKES 18 SMALL BUNS** | V

These are a beautiful and sweet addition to a winter brunch.

---

## INGREDIENTS

**FOR DOUGH:**

2 cans (5.4 ounces each) coconut cream

1 tablespoon coconut oil

1 tablespoons sugar

1 packet instant yeast

1 teaspoon vanilla extract

½ teaspoon salt

2½–3 cups all-purpose flour

**FOR FILLING:**

1 tablespoon coconut oil, softened

½ cup dark brown sugar

1½ tablespoons cinnamon

**FOR PECAN CARAMEL:**

½ cup dark brown sugar

1 tablespoon water

3 tablespoons coconut oil

1 can (5.4 ounces) coconut cream

⅔ cups chopped pecans

½ teaspoon salt

## PREPARATION

Heat coconut milk and oil in small saucepan until coconut oil is just melted. It should be just above lukewarm. If it's hotter, let it cool so you don't kill your yeast. Sprinkle sugar and yeast over warm milk and stir. Let sit for 10 minutes until yeast starts to form a small layer of bubbles. If yeast does not bubble this means it is no longer active and you'll need to start over. Add vanilla then pour into large bowl or bowl of stand mixer.

While mixing, add the flour to wet ingredients a ½ cup at a time. In dry, cold climates I find that 2½ cups of flour is perfect. If dough is still sticking to sides of bowl after 2½ cups, add flour by the tablespoon until it is very soft but not sticky. Continue to knead for 5 minutes until uniform and smooth. It will be very soft. Cover with towel and let rise in warm place for an hour.

Preheat oven to 400°F (200°C). While dough is rising, make caramel. Combine sugar and water in a small saucepan and dissolve sugar over medium heat. Add coconut oil and stir. Caramel may separate, but not to worry, it will come together when you add the coconut cream. Whisk in coconut cream and salt then bring to a boil. Boil while whisking for 2 minutes. Caramel should be smooth and uniform. It will be runny but will get thicker during baking. Pour caramel into a 8 × 11" baking dish, or a 9" cake pan works well. Sprinkle pecans over top of caramel.

Place ball of dough on a large strip of parchment paper and press (or roll out) into a ¼" thick rectangle. Spread soft coconut oil onto dough and sprinkle with brown sugar and cinnamon. With longest edge facing you, roll into a long log. Cut into 18 small rolls and place in the baking dish on top of the caramel. The rolls should be touching.

Bake for 20–25 minutes until tops are golden. Flip onto a baking sheet and lift off baking pan after a few minutes. If they are still very soft in the middle return to oven to bake for an additional 5–10 minutes.

# orange granita

**MAKES 6 CUPS** | LF | V | GF

The simplest of ingredients make this a citrus delight.

**INGREDIENTS**

5 cups freshly squeezed orange juice, strained

1 cup water

3 tablespoons maple syrup (or to taste)

**PREPARATION**

Combine all ingredients in a 9 × 13" baking dish. Place in the freezer for 3 hours. Every 30 minutes, use a fork to break up and scrape clumps of ice that begin to form.

Vitamin C is one of the most well known vitamins for a reason: it helps our skin retain elasticity, is a powerful force in neutralizing free radicals, and prevents inflammation. When citrus is consumed whole they are a tasty source of flora-enhancing fiber. Our suggestion? Squeeze in citrus at any occasion.

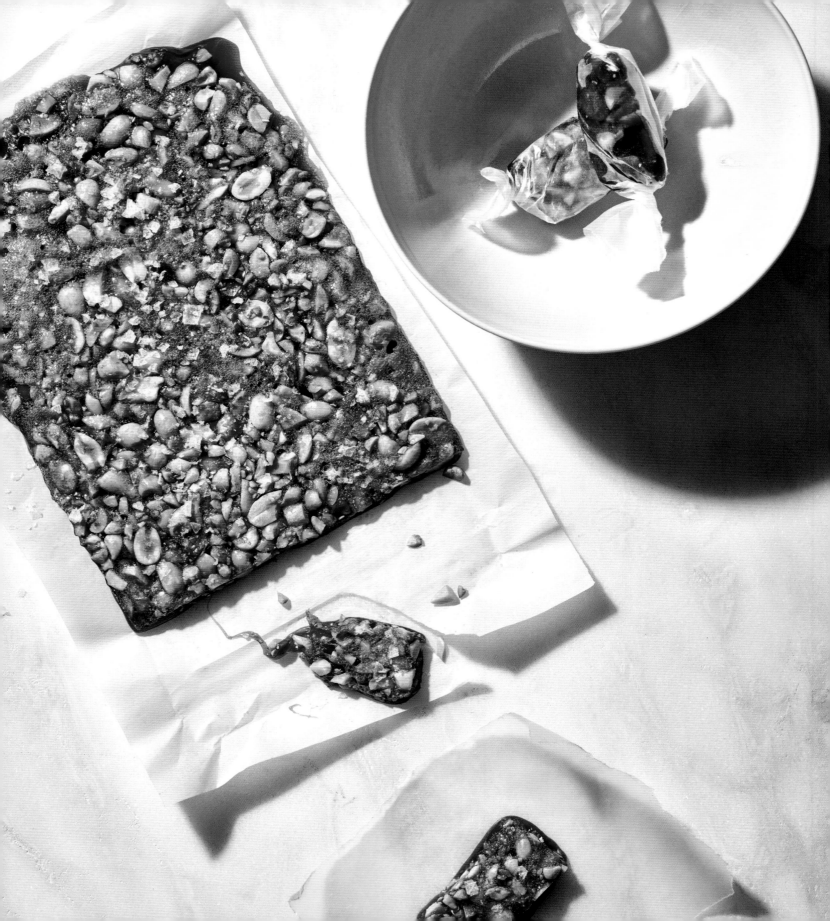

# Lala's peanut chews

**MAKES 30 (½") PIECES** | LF | V | GF

You'll need a digital or candy thermometer for this recipe so you can make sure the honey gets nice and chewy. The honey needs to reach very high temperature to caramelize and needs to be handled with caution as sugar burns can be very serious. Kids can help with wrapping the candies once they cool but the honey cooking project should be done by an adult.

**INGREDIENTS**

1 cup toasted, salted peanuts, crushed into small pieces or left whole for a chunkier texture

1 cup honey

Crunchy salt

**PREPARATION**

Line a small baking sheet with a Silpat and spread peanuts into a thin rectangle. In a small saucepan heat honey to 300°F (150°C). It will be a nice, dark amber color when it is finished. Pour hot honey over peanuts and sprinkle with crunchy salt. Let cool, cut into small rectangles, and wrap each piece in parchment or wax paper.

# turmeric golden milk

**MAKES 1 QUART** | LF | V | GF

Rooted in India's Ayurvedic tradition, golden milk is a powerful health booster. It's rich in antioxidants and fights off inflammation. If you need a little afternoon pick-me-up, give this delicious beverage a try.

### INGREDIENTS

3" piece of raw turmeric or 2 teaspoons dry turmeric

1" piece of ginger

1 cinnamon stick

A few whole cloves

A few ground peppercorns

1 quart water or favorite milk or milk substitute

Maple, honey, or sugar to taste

### PREPARATION

Simmer all ingredients except for sweetener over low heat for 20 minutes. Do not boil. Strain and sweeten to taste. Refrigerate leftovers and reheat as needed.

# ginger *or* turmeric tea

**MAKES 1 QUART** | LF | V | GF

Ginger tea can be a soothing tea throughout the day, it is warming and good for digestion. Turmeric is good for inflammation. You can make these teas separately or combine them. I like to make a quart to keep in the refrigerator and reheat as needed. If you like a spicier tea you can add more ginger and simmer for longer. If you prefer something a little more mild, you can simmer for 10 minutes.

### INGREDIENTS

3" piece of ginger, sliced into ¼" pieces and/or 3" piece fresh turmeric sliced into ¼" pieces

1 quart water

### PREPARATION

Simmer ginger and/or turmeric in water over medium heat for 20 minutes. Strain and sweeten to taste with honey or sugar.

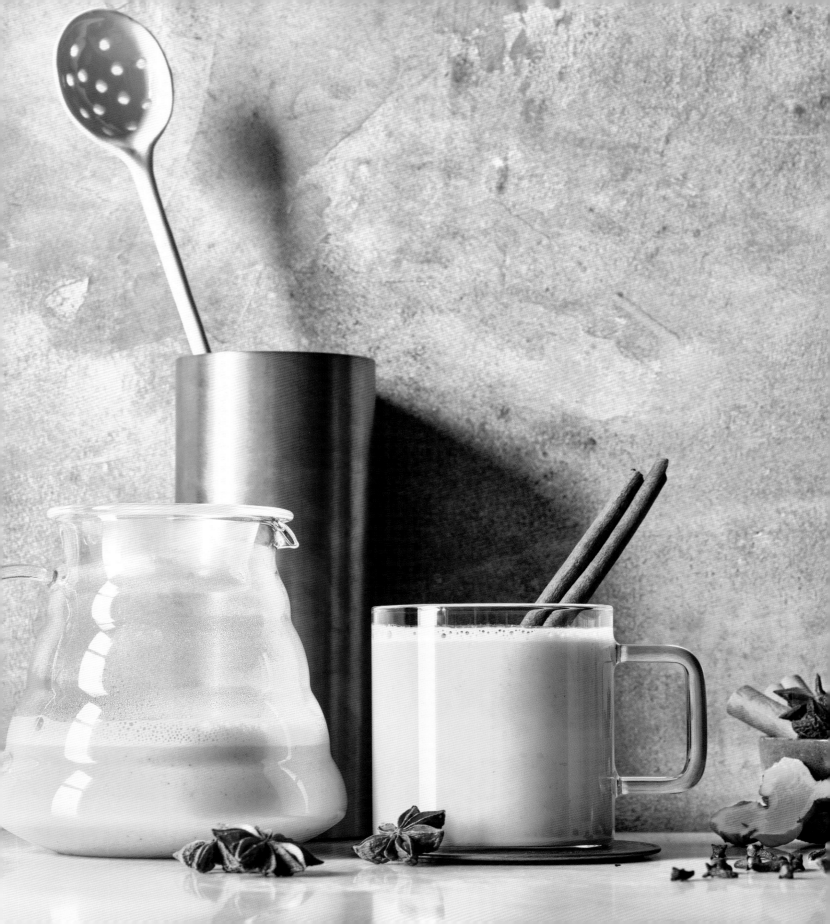

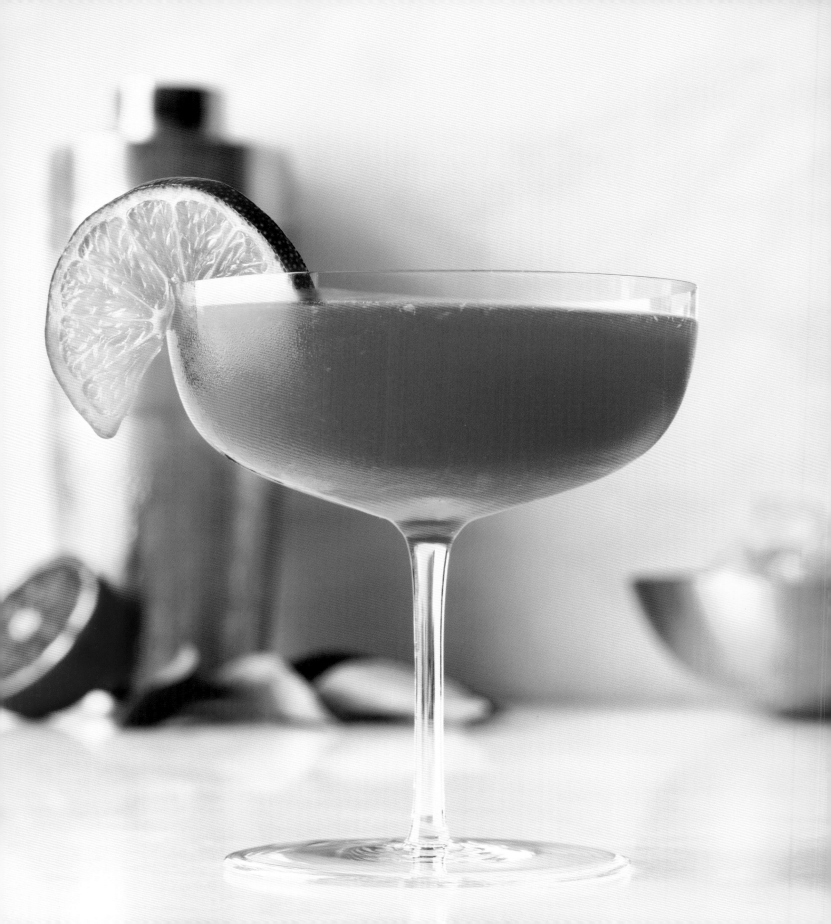

# blood orange &
# rosemary vodka cocktail

**MAKES 8 COCKTAILS** | LF | V | GF

This looks and sounds like a complicated cocktail, but it's not. Even if you're new to mixology you'll find this cocktail easy to make. The sweet tartness of the blood orange juice infused with fragrant rosemary is a palate pleaser.

## INGREDIENTS

1½ cup blood orange juice

4 springs fresh rosemary

1 cup vodka

Ice, for serving

Lime wedges, for serving

## PREPARATION

In a small saucepan, heat the blood orange juice and rosemary over low heat for 10 minutes. Allow the rosemary to infuse another 20 minutes. Remove the rosemary and discard. Allow juice to cool.

Combine rosemary-infused blood orange juice with the vodka. Pour over ice and serve with a lime wedge.

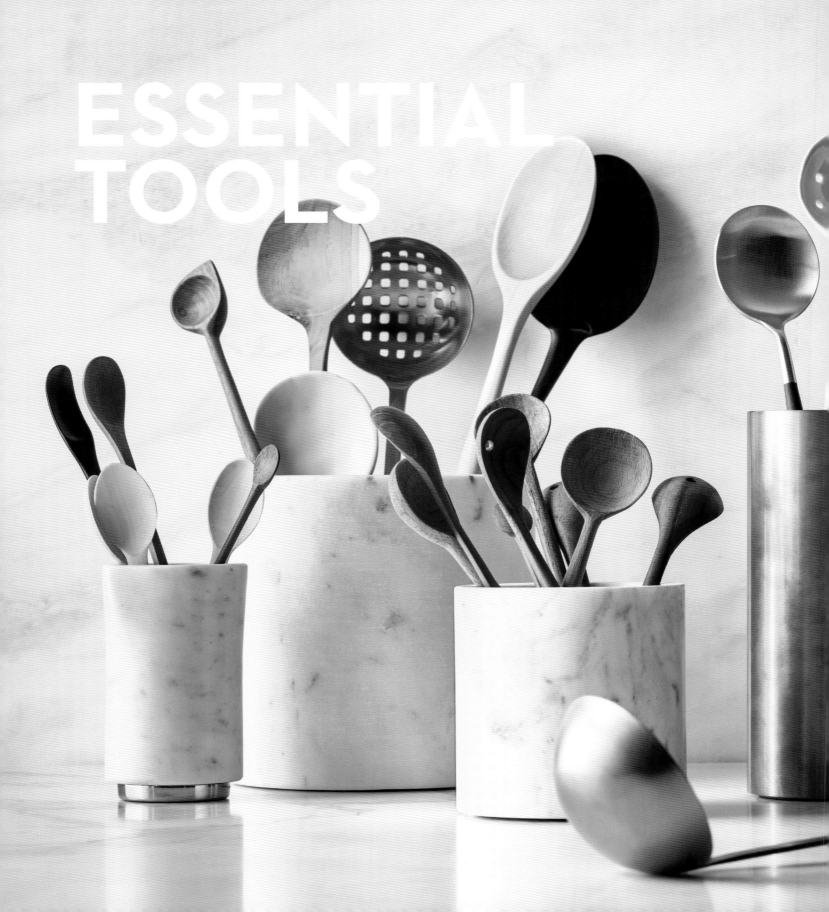

ESSENTIAL
TOOLS

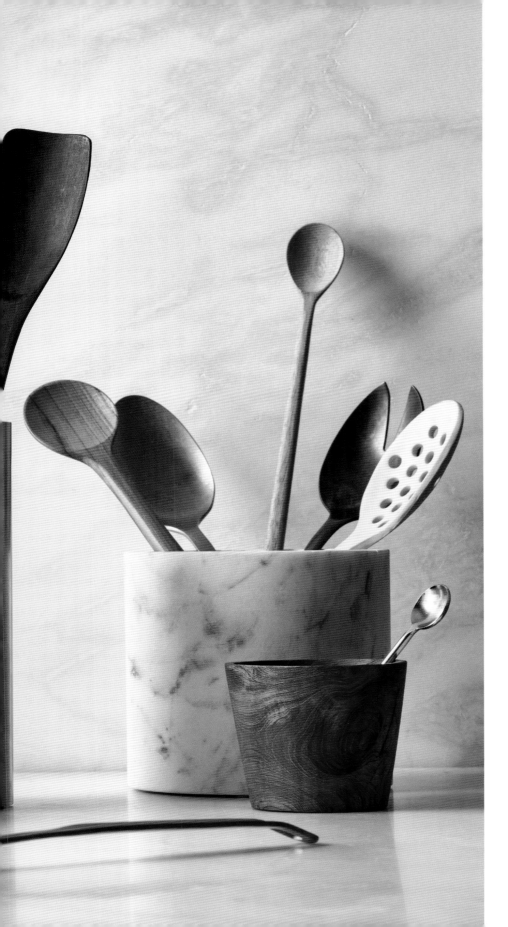

The right tools are as important as the best ingredients for cooking. At the mercy of a dull knife, that beautiful spring potato falls to pieces instead of transforming into the delicate layers that anchor your morning fritatta. Your lemon loses its zest and your chiffonade is a fraud. Here are some of the tools we just can't live without. These tools won't just bring out the best in your ingredients, they'll help you cook like a pro, or at least look like one.

**MICROPLANE** *for zesting lemons, grating garlic and ginger, finely grating Parmesan cheese. You could also use a cheese grater that has a fine grating side but a microplane is fun and a little easier for things like zesting lemons.*

**FOOD PROCESSOR** *the Cuisinart Pro Classic is a sturdy, reliable kitchen tool. KitchenAid and Breville also make good versions. Can be used for making cashew creams, quickly grating large amounts of cheese or potatoes, and making recipes like the Carrot Romesco. You can also use it for pestos and salsa verde but I find hand chopping those is a little prettier.*

**FISH SPATULA** *I use this as my go-to spatula for pretty much everything. They make a right and left handed version. I hear from my leftie friends that it does actually make a difference.*

**A SHARP CHEF'S KNIFE** *sharp knives are lovely. You can make do with dull knives but once you use sharp ones you realize how much easier and enjoyable prepping for a meal can be.*

**A COUPLE SIZES OF RUBBER SPATULAS** *for scraping out the food processor or getting the last of a batter out of a bowl. Why leave it in the dish, it's easier to clean if you fully scrape it out and then you get to enjoy eating your food rather than pouring it down the drain.*

**GLASS STORAGE DISHES AND JARS** *I am so much more apt to eat my leftovers when they are stored in an appealing dish. Plus plastic is something we can all definitely use less of for the health of our bodies and the environment.*

**PARCHMENT PAPER** *keeps you from having to scrub your sheet pans and keeps your food from sticking.*

**HALF-SIZED INDUSTRIAL STYLE SHEET PANS** *they last for a long time, stack nicely and work for everything from cookies, to oven fried chicken, to roasted potatoes.*

**ONE BIG STAINLESS STEEL SKILLET** *it is very satisfying to be able to fit dinner for 4–6 in one pan.*

**CAST IRON PAN** *not totally necessary but is a great stovetop-to-oven pan and is good looking enough to serve from.*

**DUTCH OVEN** *for making sauces and roasts. The enamel coated ones can be expensive but sometimes you can find affordable ones on sale or used and they last for ages. The well made ones become heirlooms. I have a small one from the 1930s that I adore.*

**PASTA POT** *for making pasta or large amounts of stock. A big Dutch oven could also work but pasta pots are lighter and easier to drain.*

**PAINTER'S TAPE** *for easily labeling leftovers.*

**SALAD SPINNER** *not completely necessary but I use mine all the time for greens and herbs.*

**NON-STICK PANS** *there are so many alternatives to Teflon these days. Use pans that do not have a coating with polytetrafluoroethylene (PTFE). PTFE turns toxic at high temperatures so we prefer ceramic coated non-stick pans for eggs and pancakes.*

**STAINLESS STEEL SAUCEPAN** *great for small amounts of pasta, sauces, and for cooking rice.*

**IMMERSION BLENDER** *much easier to make puréed soups right in the pot than having to pour into a traditional blender. Many have whisk/egg beater attachments as well so you don't need a separate handheld mixer.*

**HANDHELD MIXER** *for meringues and creaming butter and sugar for cakes and cookies. The stand mixer is lovely but most doughs you can knead by hand and unless you are an avid baker they aren't necessary (though I do love them).*

**A COUPLE DIFFERENT SIZES OF CUTTING BOARDS** *smaller ones for cutting up something for a snack, a larger one for making dinner. I like bamboo—they are easy to clean and eco-friendly, just don't let them sit in the sink or they will warp and get moldy.*

**PIZZA CUTTER** *because pizza.*

**DIGITAL THERMOMETER** *many digital ones can be used for testing meat as well as have a high enough temperature gauge for candy making.*

**SPIRILIZER** *for making vegetable noodles for salads and pasta substitutes.*

**MESH VEGETABLE BAGS** *not necessary but they are cheap and it is another way to cut back on the amount of plastic you use.*

**CHEESE CLOTH** *for broths and nut milks.*

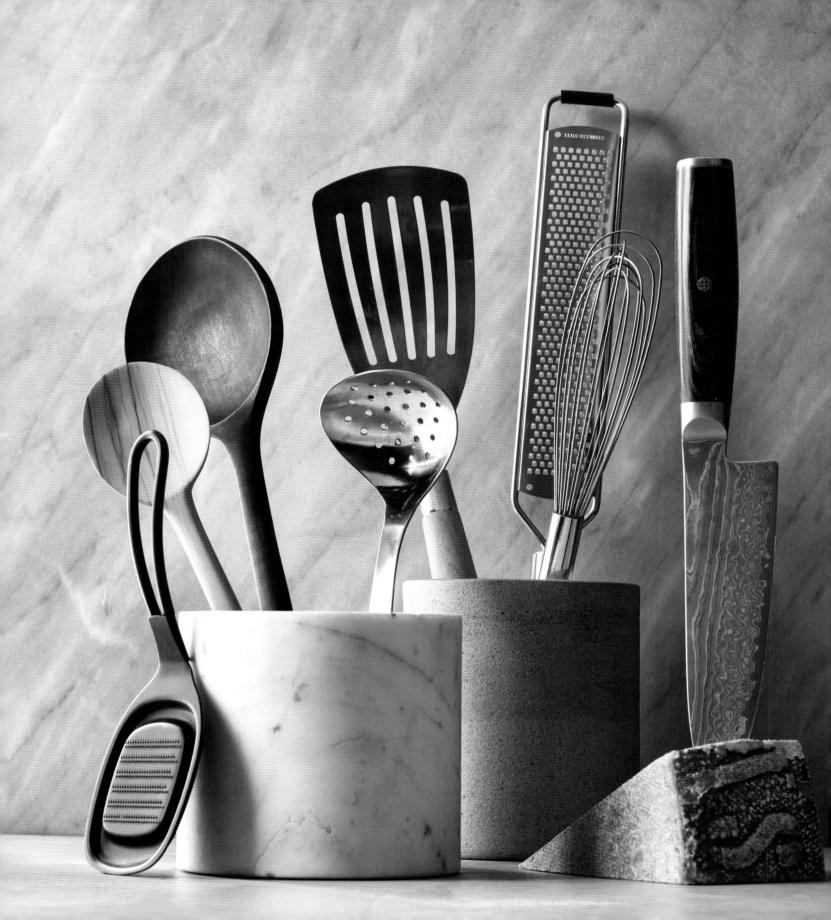

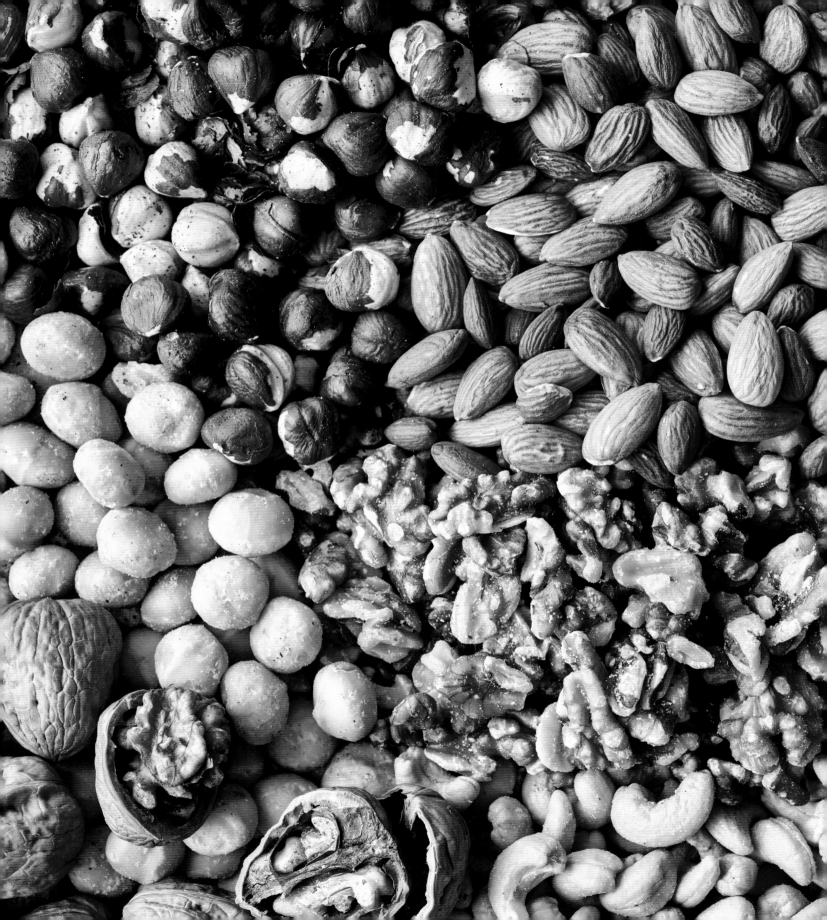

# COOKING FOR LEFTOVERS & FOOD STORAGE GUIDELINES

*When hunger strikes, it can be make or break for your microbiome health. Reach for something microbiome-healthy and you're satiated and energized. Grab something that throws your system out of whack and, well, you know how the story ends.*

*To avoid those microbiome-wrecking moments, we always cook enough to have leftovers on hand. Since they are such an important way to maintain SIBO health and balance, we've compiled a few tips and guidelines for safe storage.*

---

### USE SEE-THROUGH CONTAINERS

If you can't see it, you probably won't eat it, so use see-through containers for easy scanning.

### USE PAINTER'S TAPE TO LABEL

This is a trick used by chefs and restaurants to keep track of prepared items. Use painter's tape and a permanent marker to mark containers with what's inside and what date it was cooked. This goes for restaurant leftovers as well.

### KEEP LEFTOVERS UP TOP

Keep prepared foods at the top of the refrigerator, where they're in sight and away from any possible drips from other items. (Another good rule of thumb is to store raw meats double wrapped and on bottom shelves.)

### STORE LEFTOVERS QUICKLY

Leftovers should be in the refrigerator as soon as possible, within two hours or one hour if it's 90°F (32°C) or above. Bacteria grow in temperatures between 40°F–140°F (4°C–60°C), so getting them into refrigeration as soon as possible—not letting them cool on the counter or stovetop—is key.

### KEEP YOUR REFRIGERATOR BELOW 40°F (4°C)

Most people do not keep their refrigerator cool enough. A temperature of below 40°F (4°C) is needed to keep bacterial growth at bay. Use a refrigerator thermometer to ensure yours is at a safe-for-storage temperature.

### KEEP IT COOL FOR TRAVEL

Just like leaving foods on the countertop, toting perishables in a lunchbox or in the car for extended times can lead to bacteria growth. If you are on a road trip, tailgating or picnicking, keep meals and snacks in a well insulated cooler with ice or cold packs.

### 3–4 DAYS (REFRIGERATOR) SHELF LIFE

If stored quickly and at the correct temperatures, you can expect leftovers to keep for 3–4 days. Marking the date will help you keep track, since at the early stages of growth, bacteria don't typically change the look or taste of food but can be present in numbers that can cause illness. Never taste your food to check, even a small taste can make you sick. When in doubt, throw it out.

### THREE SAFE WAYS TO THAW

Thawing on the countertop isn't safe—foods may quickly reach the 40°F (4°C) threshold of bacteria growth. When thawing foods, use one of these three methods:

- **REFRIGERATOR** *As long as the temperature inside the refrigerator is below 40°F (4°C), foods will safely, if somewhat slowly, thaw. Foods thawed in the refrigerator can be refrigerated for two days before cooking; 3–5 days for steaks, lamb, and pork.*

- **COLD WATER** *Submerge the item in cold water, changing the water every 30 minutes. Make sure items are sealed in a bag or container as any water or air could contain bacteria. Cook or reheat immediately after thawing.*

- **MICROWAVE** *Make sure that the food rotates during heating or thawing as one area may be warm and the other cold.*

### RE-HEAT TO 165°F (74°C)

If reheating or cooking from frozen, it's important that food reaches a safe temperature of 165°F (74°C). Microwaved food should sit for one minute before testing. The exterior is often a few degrees warmer than the core so insert the food thermometer well into the middle of the item for an accurate, and safe, reading.

# THE SIBO FOOD LIST

*Cooking for SIBO and microbiome balance is easy...once you get the hang of it. The key thing to remember is that it's not about having to give up all the foods that you love. The following table lists the foods that are healthy (green) and not healthy (red).*

# FOODS TO EAT.

## CARBOHYDRATES

*It's important for SIBO patients to be mindful when it comes to carbohydrate portions at each meal. Aim to limit carbohydrates to 1 serving per meal.*

Bagel (rye, sourdough or plain; limit to ½ bagel)

Bread crumbs

Bread, French

Bread, Italian

Bread, potato

Bread, refined, white or wheat

Bread, rye

Cereals: refined (Rice Krispies, Original Special K, cornflakes)

Cornmeal

Cornstarch

Couscous

Crackers, refined (such as Rustic Bakery, La Panzanella)

Cream of wheat

Dumpling wrappers

Gnocchi

Noodles, egg

Noodles, udon

Orzo

Panko (regular and gluten-free)

Pasta

Pasta (gluten-free made from white rice, corn, or almond flour)

Phyllo dough

Polenta

Popchips

Popcorn

Potato flour

Quinoa

Rice (white, sushi, paella, jasmine)

Rice cakes (made from white rice only)

Rye flour

Seitan

Sourdough bread

Tortillas (corn or flour)

Tortilla chips

## PROTEIN/MEAT

Bacon: w/o nitrates and HFCS

Beef

Eggs

Fish

Game

Lamb

Organ meats

Poultry

Seafood

Seitan

## VEGETABLES

Avocado

Beets

Capers

Caper berries

Carrots

Celeriac

Celery: peel the skin; limit, best to use to flavor soups and stews.

# FOODS TO EAT. *(continued)*

Chives

Corn

Cucumbers (Persian cucumbers are less gassy but all types are acceptable.)

Eggplant

Endive (in small amounts)

English peas

Fennel (root only)

Garlic (cooked is typically better tolerated)

Green beans

Greens: arugula, kale, and spinach are best. Hold off initially on butter lettuce and romaine as they are often not tolerated as well.

Horseradish

Jicama

Leek

Mushrooms

Olives

Onion (in small amounts; cooked is typically better tolerated)

Parsnips

Peas (green, in small amounts)

Peppers (bell, chili)

Potatoes

Pumpkin

Radicchio

Rhubarb

Rutabaga (root only, not leaves)

Scallion (green parts only)

Seaweed

Shallot (in small amounts; cooked is typically better tolerated)

Squash

Sweet potato

Swiss chard

Tomatillo

Tomato

Turnips

Water chestnut

Yam

Yucca

Zucchini

## FRUIT

*Fruit is an important part of a healthy, balanced diet. When eating to manage SIBO, one serving at a time is recommended. Please note, dried fruit is not suggested, even when made from an allowed fruit.*

Apricots, fresh

Blackberries

Blueberries

Boysenberries

Cantaloupe (limit to one cup)

Cherries

Cranberries

Dragon fruit

Grapefruit

Grapes

Guava

Honeydew (limit to one cup)

Kiwi

Lemons

Limes

Mango

Nectarine

Okra

Oranges

Papaya

Passion fruit

Peaches

Persimmon

Pineapple

Plum

Pomegranate

Raspberries

Strawberries

Tamarillo

Tangerines

Watermelon (limit to one cup)

# FOODS TO EAT. *(continued)*

## DAIRY

Butter (small amounts)

Cheese, most aged and hard varieties, like Parmesan, Cheddar, Manchego, and Gruyère

Dairy-alternative milks such as almond milk, rice milk, coconut milk, oat milk, and hemp milk

Ghee

Lactose-free cottage cheese

Lactose-free milk

## NUTS & SEEDS

Almonds

Cashews

Chestnuts

Coconut

Hazelnuts

Hemp seeds

Macadamia nuts

Nut butters

Peanuts

Pecans

Pine nuts

Pistachios

Pumpkin seeds

Sesame seeds

Sunflower seeds

Walnuts

## HERBS, SPICES, & SEASONINGS

*Both dried and fresh versions are SIBO-friendly*

Basil

Bay leaf

Cardamom

Cayenne

Chamomile

Chervil

Chili flakes

Chili powder

Chives

Cilantro

Cinnamon

Cumin

Curry powder

Dill

Everything spice

Fennel seed

Ginger

Garlic powder

Herbs de Provence

Hibiscus

Kaffir lime

Lemon verbena

Lemongrass

Mint

Mustard, dry

Nettle

Nutritional yeast

Onion powder

Oregano

Paprika

Parsley

Pepper

Poultry seasoning

Rosemary

Saffron

Sage

Salt

Sumac

Tarragon

Thyme

Turmeric

Vanilla bean

Wasabi powder

## BAKING, SWEETS, & SWEETENERS

*Note: table sugar is absorbed higher up in the GI tract before the bacteria can feed off of it.*

Active dry yeast

Agar flakes

All-purpose flour

Almond flour

Aspartame

Baking powder

Baking soda

Chocolate, bittersweet

Chocolate, dark

Chocolate, semisweet

Cocoa powder

Coffee instant/
espresso granules

Corn flour

Cream of tartar

Equal Sugar Substitute

Honey (in small amounts)

Maple syrup

Orange blossom water

Pomegranate molasses

Sorbet (one scoop maximum)

Sugar (cane, turbinado, caster)

Vanilla extract

Vanilla powder

## CONDIMENTS

Avocado oil

Barbeque sauce w/o HFCS
(such as FODY, Tessamae's)

Canola oil

Chili paste

Coconut aminos

Coconut oil

Cornichons

Fish sauce

Ginger, pickled

Gochujang

Grapeseed oil

Jam
(made from approved fruits)

Ketchup w/o HFCS (such as
Simply Heinz, Sir Kensington's,
Annie's Organic, Woodstock
Organic, or Primal Kitchen)

Kuzu

Mayonnaise

Mustard

Olive oil

Relish

Sesame oil

Soy sauce

Sriracha

Sunflower oil

Tomato and pasta sauce
(Rao's sensitive formula is
suggested for those who cannot
tolerate onion and garlic)

Tomato paste

Vegetable oil

Vinegar

Worcestershire sauce
(Lord Sandy's Vegan)

## BEVERAGES

Broth

Coffee

Juice of approved fruits and
vegetables (small portions)

Seltzer/carbonated beverages
(without HFCS)

Teas

Water

## ALCOHOL

Beer (note: less hoppy beers
are more likely to be tolerated)

Bourbon

Brandy

Champagne

Gin

Grappa

Port

Rum

Sake

Sherry

Tequila

Vermouth

Vodka

Whiskey/scotch

Wine (all red and white varieties)

# FOODS TO AVOID.

## CARBOHYDRATES

*It's important for SIBO patients to be mindful when it comes to carbohydrate portions at each meal. Aim to limit carbohydrates to 1 serving per meal.*

Bran

Bread, multigrain

Bread, whole wheat

Brown rice

Buckwheat flour

Bulgur wheat

Cereals, whole wheat

Farrow

Flour, multigrain

Oat bran

Oatmeal

Pasta, whole wheat

Soba noodles

Spelt flour

## VEGETABLES

Alfalfa sprouts

Artichoke

Asparagus

Bamboo shoots

Bean sprouts

Bok choy

Broccoli

Brussels sprouts

Cabbage

Cauliflower

Chicory root

Edamame

Radish

Snow peas

Sugar snap peas

Tamarind

## FRUIT

*Fruit is an important part of a healthy, balanced diet. When eating to manage SIBO, one serving at a time is recommended. Please note, dried fruit is not suggested, even when made from an allowed fruit.*

Apples

Apricots, dried

Bananas

Dates

Dried fruits

Figs

Fruit-juice concentrates

Monk fruit

Pears

Prunes

Raisins

# FOODS TO AVOID. *(continued)*

## DAIRY

Cheese (soft, not aged)

Cream cheese*

Milk

Soy milk

Yogurt**

*Lactose-free cream cheese and lactose-free sour cream made by Green Valley has live cultures. Patients who have been symptom-free for 3 months can enjoy these on occasion.*
**Lactose-free yogurt is not suggested for those with SIBO due to the live cultures present.*

## LEGUMES

Beans (most varieties)

Black beans

Butter beans

Cannellini beans

Chickpea/garbanzo beans

Fava beans

Hummus

Kidney beans

Lentils

Lima beans

Navy beans

Pinto beans

Soy products
(in meat alternatives)

Soybeans

Tempeh

Tofu

White beans

## MEAT

Marinated Steak
(i.e. from a steakhouse;
marinades have HFCS)

## NUTS & SEEDS

Chia seeds

Flax seeds

## CONDIMENTS

Barbeque sauce with HFCS

Cooking oils with additives

Plum sauce

Sweet and sour sauce

## BAKING, SWEETS, & SWEETENERS

Agave

Aspertame

Equal

Erythritol

High-fructose corn syrup

Lactose (in dairy)

Mannitol (sugar alcohol)

Monk fruit extract

Sacharin

Sorbitol (sugar alcohol)

Splenda

Stevia

Sucralose

Xylitol (sugar alcohol)

## BEVERAGES

Drinks with HFCS

Soda

# RECIPE INDEX

# RECIPE INDEX *(continued)*

# INDEX

# INDEX *(continued)*

# INDEX *(continued)*

# INDEX *(continued)*

# INDEX *(continued)*

*Let food be thy medicine & medicine be thy food...*

*— Hippocrates*

First printed in April 2022

Printed in China

10 9 8 7 6 5 4 3 2 1          22 23 24 25

ISBN-13: 978-1-57284-307-3
ISBN-10: 1-57284-307-1
eISBN-13: 978-1-57284-857-3
eISBN-10: 1-57284-857-X

Library of Congress Cataloging-in-Publication Data is available from the Library of Congress

Surrey is an imprint of Agate Publishing. Agate books are available in bulk at discount prices. For more information, visit agatepublishing.com.

## CREDITS

### Krystyna

A busy mom of three, Krystyna's journey to identify her microbiome problems and develop her treatment took several years, numerous dead ends, and involved experts from multiple disciplines. Krystyna's determination to continue enjoying food with family and friends, while establishing and maintaining better microbiome health was the inspiration and guiding spirit for this book. Here she shares her love of cooking, recipes, and "hacks" that keep eating fun, and her microbiome in balance.

### Robin

Robin Berlin is a Registered Dietitian who has worked in the Los Angeles area for over 15 years. Her focus is on diet, wellness, lifestyle, and movement. Robin works with clients from around the globe and collaborates with leading physicians with expertise in GI, Cardiology, Oncology, and other sub-specialties. As someone with a history of SIBO, Robin has studied and focused on the microbiome and gut health for years. With a personal passion and a professional commitment, she instills a sense of hope to those affected by GI disorders and teaches them how to cook and eat so they can enjoy food without fear.

### Misti

Misti Boettiger is a cook, creative problem solver, and relationship-building storyteller fascinated by sustainable food practices and collaborative design. Misti loves blending her professional chops with personal improvisation to create new dishes or reinvent traditional favorites to meet the tastes or dietary needs of modern palates. Misti approaches food without hard and fast rules, only the belief that you can't fake quality ingredients or cooking that comes from the heart.

### Authors:

Krystyna Houser
Robin Berlin

### Executive Test Chef:

Misti Boettiger

Produced by Exquisite Corp.
Creative Director: Richard Klein
Account Director: Erin Posey
Editor: Jenny Shears
Associate Art Director: Alec Nikolajevich
Photographer: Leigh Beisch
Food Styling: Emily Caneer
Assistant: Jillian Mosley
Prop Styling: Glenn Jenkins